Good Bacteria for Healthy Skin

NURTURE YOUR SKIN MICROBIOME WITH PRE- AND PROBIOTICS FOR CLEAR AND LUMINOUS SKIN

PAULA SIMPSON

ULYSSES PRESS

Published in the United States by:
ULYSSES PRESS
P.O. Box 3440
Berkeley, CA 94703
www.ulyssespress.com

ISBN: 978-1-61243-930-3
Library of Congress Control Number: 2019942126

Printed in Canada by Marquis Book Printing
10 9 8 7 6 5 4 3 2 1

Acquisitions editor: Casie Vogel
Managing editor: Claire Chun
Project editor: Claire Sielaff
Editor: Lauren Harrison
Proofreader: Renee Rutledge
Indexer: Sayre Van Young
Front cover design: Raquel Castro
Cover photos: © VICUSCHKA/shutterstock.com
Interior design: what!design @ whatweb.com
Interior art: pages 24, 25 © NeutronStar8/shutterstock.com; pages 67, 78 © yoyoai/
    shutterstock.com

*I want to dedicate this book to my husband Kevin
and my daughter Sierra. Your ongoing love, support and amazing
sense of humor makes each day joyful and bright, even amongst
the most challenging times. I'm grateful for you both.*

For my dad and brother, with love and fond memories.

Contents

〜〜〜

Introduction. 1

Living in Symbiosis 2

Advancing Science. 2

CHAPTER 1: *The Gut-Brain-Skin Axis* 5

Your Gut and Skin. 8

Your Brain and Skin. 9

Quick Nutrition Tips to Combat Stress
(and Save Your Skin) 13

CHAPTER 2: *The Skin Microbiome—*
the Missing Link for Healthy Skin?. 19

Structure, Function and Importance of the
Skin Microbiome 21

Skin Structure. 23

What Constitutes a Healthy Skin Microbiota? 25

The Key Players 27

Avoiding Dysbiosis 29

CHAPTER 3: *Lifestyle and the Skin Microbiome*. . 34

We All Emit a "Biome Cloud" 35

The Stratum Corneum and Skin Microbiome
Working Together 36

Environmental Factors Affecting the Skin Microbiome 38

Challenging the "Hygiene Hypothesis" 41

Topicals and Cosmetics. 45

Diet. 47

CHAPTER 4: *Skin Conditions Associated
with the Skin Microbiome* **49**

Introduction to Probiotics and Prebiotics 50

Microbes, Pre- and Probiotics, and Chronic
Skin Conditions 53

CHAPTER 5: *What You Should Know about
Pre- and Probiotics* **64**

Common Probiotics 65

Probiotics—How They Work and What to Look
for on a Label 69

Prebiotics. 75

CHAPTER 6: *Microbe-Friendly Nutrition* **85**

How Good Nutrition Promotes Healthy Skin. 86

You Are What You Consume, Metabolize and Flourish. 87

Beautify Your Skin Biome with Microbe-Friendly
Nutrition. 88

Microbe-Friendly Nutrition—Dietary Considerations. 89

The Macronutrients. 91

Flourish with Fermented Foods. 96

Pre- and Probiotic Supplements 103

CHAPTER 7: *Microbe-Friendly Skincare* 107

Natural Elements for the Skin Microbiome 110

Nourishing Mask with Probiotics and Honey 113

What to Look for in Probiotic Skincare 115

Beautifying Your Biome from the Outside 119

CHAPTER 8: *Putting It Together: The Beauty Biome Lifestyle* 122

Beautify Your Skin Biome—The Plan. 124

Biome Beauty Nutrition Essentials. 125

Restock Your Kitchen 127

Start Your Day Biome-Friendly and Beauty-Infused. 128

Biome Beauty Meals. 130

Juices, Broths and Teas 132

Biome Beauty Skincare Plan 133

Soothing and Moisturizing Probiotic Mask 134

CHAPTER 9: *Biome Beauty Dietary Recipes*. 140

Quinoa with Red Peppers 141

Baked Salmon with Pesto. 142

"Get Your Greens" Salad with Beets and
Avocado-Miso Dressing 143

Savory Roasted Chickpeas 144

Kimchi Omelet Anytime of the Day 145

Balsamic Vinaigrette Dressing. 145

Grilled Salmon and Vegetables 146

Bone Broth 147

Biome-Purifying Tonic 148

Biome-Purifying and Detox Broth .149

Fresh Juices 150
Luminous Skin and Antioxidant Smoothie 150
Clarifying Smoothie 151
Fortifying Skin, Hair and Nails Smoothie. 152
"Glo" and Go Smoothie 152

Conclusion 154

Notes 156

Index 175

Acknowledgments 182

About the Author 184

Introduction

〰〰

Let's talk about dirt. I mean real dirt. From what makes up the earth and soil to objects, humans, animals and the air we breathe. Beyond what we can see with the naked eye lies a codependent community of microorganisms that are constantly evolving in conjunction with their environment.

I'm talking about germs. Over the last 20 years, scientific research has evolved and is perhaps beginning to change the way we think about germs. These microorganisms (bacteria, fungi and even parasites) that occupy the human body may in some cases be more helpful to our health than harmful. According to scientists, "microbes" should no longer be regarded as the "bad guys" because they're not all bad; rather, a vast majority of them work as helpers to protect us from harmful pathogens and keep our health in balance.[1]

Moreover, an excessive use of antibiotics and unhealthy Western diets pose a serious threat to the composition and balance of the microorganisms. These factors weaken the homeostasis of the microbiome (the full collection of microbes and their genes) and overall health of the human body. This new way of thinking has

the potential to disrupt our modern Western lifestyle, from how we eat and take care of our skin to our compulsion to maintain overly sterile environments.

LIVING IN SYMBIOSIS

Think about this: We aren't solitary beings living in isolation; rather we are moving ecosystems adapting to our changing environment, living in symbiosis. To be efficient, a symbiotic relationship needs ongoing equilibrium, which is the result of long years of coevolution. Bacteria were the first active things on the planet, with other beings living and evolving with them for hundreds of millions of years. Now microbes are essential for many organisms' basic tasks, including nourishment, reproduction and protection.

ADVANCING SCIENCE

With the advancement of DNA sequencing techniques, researchers can now describe the diversity of microbes residing on and within our bodies. These microbial communities inhabiting us have collectively been called "the human microbiome." This field of study received a great boost in 2007 when the National Institutes of Health initiated the Human Microbiome Project (HMP) with the intent of surveying and characterizing the microbes that reside in different parts of the body. Today, with the groundwork prepared by those earlier explanatory studies, we are able to uncover the intimate relationships that microbes share with us (the host) and the influences they have on our health.[2]

But what comes with this fascinating new science is a lot of confusion and oversimplification. Not a day goes by that we don't read something about the benefits of "good bacteria" for our mental

and physical well-being (more formally known as the "gut-brain-skin axis," which we'll talk about further in Chapter 1) or why we should be consuming probiotic-rich foods and supplements and applying them to our skin. The health market, and more recently the skin- and haircare markets, are being flooded with products touting these bacteria as the missing link between optimal health and natural beauty.

My natural curiosity guided me to write this book in hopes of dismantling the misconceptions and overgeneralization about the skin microbiome. As a biochemist and nutritionist, I am a big supporter of pre- and probiotics from diet and supplements for my clients. As a key organ for elimination, the digestive system is how we absorb macro- and micronutrients, as well as expel toxins and waste. It is the foundation of our immune system. When your digestion isn't healthy, your total health suffers. But when the gut microbiome is balanced and thriving, you digest and absorb nutrients efficiently while excreting toxins and pathogens before they are absorbed into the bloodstream. We will talk more about this in Chapter 1, but Dr. Nigma Talib does a fabulous job summarizing the connection between our gut and skin health in her book *Younger Skin Starts in the Gut*.

Because I have also spent much of my professional time collaborating with medical experts, researching and formulating with companies to create natural health products focused on skin health and beauty, I was intrigued by the evidence coming out around the skin microbiome and its potential impact on the skin's health and appearance. Along with the digestive system, liver, kidneys and lungs, the skin also functions as an organ of elimination and is the one most exposed to stressors from our environment. The skin microbiome is the most complex, dynamic and sophisticated ecosystems throughout the body. When this ecosystem is balanced

and thriving, skin is even toned, moist and absent of blemishes or redness.

I wrote this book to make this complex topic more easily understood, to provide a scientifically sound yet approachable overview of the "prettier" side of germs and to help reveal your healthiest skin possible.

I hope you enjoy it,

Paula

CHAPTER 1

The Gut-Brain-Skin Axis

~~~

The human microbiome, a term proposed by the well-known geneticist Joshua Lederberg, refers to all those microbes that are found in and on human beings. We as humans are mostly microbes—more than 100 trillion of them live inside or on our bodies. They outnumber human cells 10 to 1. The microbiome may weigh as much as 5 pounds and comprises 99 percent of the cells on the body. These bacteria help us digest our food, produce certain vitamins, support the immune system and protect the body from foreign invaders. An unbalanced microbiome, a term known as "dysbiosis," has been connected with certain autoimmune diseases such as diabetes, rheumatoid arthritis, muscular dystrophy and fibromyalgia. Chronic dysbiosis of the gut microbiome, for example, has been implicated in conditions including leaky gut syndrome, inflammation and weight gain, and it also influences the health and appearance of our skin.[3]

Your body and brain are in constant communication. For example, there is continual interaction between the gut, its microbiome and the brain to regulate a multitude of metabolic, immune, endocrine and nervous system processes. Studies show that mental stress can alter gut microbiota, and to some degree gut microbiota has the ability to influence stress-related behaviors.[4]

Your skin is also a prominent target organ for numerous neuro-signals that may have a profound impact on your skin health. This "brain-skin connection" has inspired researchers in the inseparable fields of neurology, microbiology, genetics, biochemistry and dermatology to learn more about this sophisticated signaling network. If you've ever heard of the saying "You are what you eat," this also holds true for the gut-brain-skin axis that regularly adapts and changes based on diet, lifestyle and the environment we live in.[5] So, you could say instead, "You are not only what you eat, but also what you live in."

MICROBES AND YOU: QUICK FACTS

* A microbe is a living organism too small to be seen by the naked eye.

* "Microbes" is a general term used to describe different types of life forms including bacteria, fungi, algae, protozoa and viruses.

* The microbiome is recognized as the collective genomes of the microbes that live inside and on the human body. We have about 10 times as many microbial cells as human cells.

* We are exposed to microbes at birth, and they continue to flourish and diversify based on our environment and climate, age, gender, diet and

lifestyle. Our genetic makeup can also have an indirect effect on our microbiome.

* Microbes are diverse, and there is a trend for certain microbes to survive in and prefer different body sites over others, such as moist versus dry skin.

* Within their ecosystem, microbes coexist and strive to maintain a state of "symbiosis," or balance with their host. They are essential in protecting us, providing nourishment and communicating with our immune system to maintain optimal health and balance.

* When microbes become imbalanced, this is known as "dysbiosis" and is believed to be a factor in the progression of certain diseases and conditions.[6]

Think about it like this: How you react to stressful situations, what you consume, and where and how you live every day have a profound effect on the state of your gut and skin microbiome. Those external stressors (either psychological or environmental) have the ability to change the gut microflora, reducing their diversity and balance and stressing normal digestive processes. This "stressed ecosystem" weakens the gut barrier, allowing harmful endotoxins and byproducts to pass more easily through the intestinal wall and enter the bloodstream, a condition known as leaky gut syndrome. Once these endotoxins enter blood circulation, they stimulate a cascade of pro-inflammatory reactions and unstable reactive cells (referred to as a state of oxidative stress) that have the ability to attack healthy skin tissue and alter the balance and health of the skin microbiome. This complex cycle includes a series of signals and reactions from neurotransmitters, hormones, metabolites and microorganisms that work collectively as a whole system. Because

all of these things are interconnected, if just one part of this complex community becomes unbalanced or off-kilter, the whole system is affected. Truly amazing!

YOUR GUT AND SKIN

The general well-being of your body depends on three basic elements:

1. The quality of nutrients you eat.

2. How well these nutrients are digested and absorbed.

3. How well toxins and wastes are neutralized and removed.

When we eat nutrient-deficient and processed diets, i.e., the typical Western diet, dietary contaminants cause "body burden." This strains the eliminative organs (the liver, kidneys, digestion, lungs and skin) and circulates toxins to peripheral organs, fat tissue and the skin.

The human digestive system is a complex system that is composed of functionally distinct regions: the oral cavity, stomach, small intestine and colon. For example, the mouth is home to at least 6 billion microorganisms, while the gastric microflora is slightly more acidic and less diverse, as are the small intestine and colon microbiomes. The gut microbiome performs significant functions for the health of the human body, including synthesis of vitamins, decomposition of chemicals and nutrients, support of fat metabolism, outcompeting pathogens, and the balance and development of the immune system.[7]

The gut microbiota also produces metabolites, neurotransmitters and hormones that can enter the bloodstream and modify the

skin. Likewise, the skin creates a selection of chemicals that could modify the gut, such as vitamin D. As mentioned earlier, when there is a leaky gut barrier or gut dysbiosis (microbial imbalance), contaminants and harmful bacteria from the gut pass through to the bloodstream. These harmful bacteria and endotoxins have a domino effect on the cells, creating a pro-inflammatory environment and oxidative stress in the body with consequences for the skin. The use of prebiotics and probiotics has been shown to help stabilize the gut microbiome and ultimately have a positive effect on the skin, including improving conditions like skin aging, acne, atopic dermatitis and rosacea.[8]

HEALTHY GUT MICROFLORA

* Detoxify and protect the body from harmful bacteria (before it's absorbed into bloodstream)
* Support immunity
* Encourage nutrient bioavailability
* Balance pH in the intestine
* Support and balance skin microflora

YOUR BRAIN AND SKIN

No question, stress is a part of our daily lives, and we all know how detrimental it can be to our health. It aggravates many ailments, like headaches and brain fog, digestive upset, weight gain, cardiovascular disease, depressed immunity, increased blood pressure, blood sugar problems, skin wrinkles and emotional sensitivity.

Since 2006, the American Psychological Association's Stress in America annual survey has examined sources of stress and its

impact on the health and well-being of Americans. The results of the 2017 poll showed a statistically significant increase in stress for the first time since the survey was conducted in 2006. The percentage of Americans who reported experiencing at least one symptom of stress over the past month rose from 71 percent in 2016 to 80 percent in 2017. It is estimated that 75 to 90 percent of visits to primary care physicians are related to stress.[9]

Apart from the acute "fight or flight" stress response, habitual stress is harmful to our health because it strains the hypothalamic-pituitary-adrenal (HPA) axis, our central stress response system, which links the central nervous and endocrine systems. When we experience psychological or even physical stress, the brain activates a series of hormone-releasing reactions through the HPA axis and stimulates the production of reactive stress hormones, which remain elevated over time. So when you are chronically stressed, these hormones work like a car in overdrive—it will eventually run out of gas, a condition we know as burnout or adrenal fatigue.

Have you ever noticed that when you're dealing with more stress than usual, your skin reacts too? It's no coincidence. Scientists refer to this connection as the "brain-skin" axis in the study of the effects of psychological stress on the skin. Acne, eczema and atopic dermatitis have been found to be more active during times of emotional stress. Cortisol is a major stress hormone that has been found to be chronically elevated in those who suffer with acne. According to research, people who are prone to acne are more likely to suffer from stress and anxiety.[10] Also, in a recent study conducted on medical students, increased psychological stress significantly correlated with greater acne severity, with researchers citing the hyper activity of the HPA axis as a primary cause.[11] Additionally, individuals who are prone to acne are more

likely to experience gastrointestinal distress due to an imbalanced gut microflora with reduced levels of good gut bacteria.[12] You can see how all of these studies just emphasize the power of the human microbiome and codependence of the brain, gut and skin.

When we are stressed, the following reactions may occur and impact the skin:

* The corticotropin-releasing hormone (CRH) is stimulated and acts as a central coordinator for neuroendocrine and behavioral responses to stress. CRH also stimulates sebum production and pro-inflammatory byproducts, which contribute to acne.

* Cortisol is released from the adrenal glands and changes receptor activity in the skin cells that produce sebum, promoting oily and congested skin. Cortisol also affects blood sugar levels and reduces insulin sensitivity, which can break down healthy skin collagen.

* Skin mast cells (regulators in inflammatory, hypersensitivity and allergic reactions) become more responsive and release chemicals that promote inflammation.

* Normal skin cellular renewal cycles are impaired.

* The skin microbiota become less diverse and more unbalanced, increasing "bad" bacteria overload. This imbalance of the microbiota lowers skin pH, increases skin redness and sensitivity, and promotes congestion and blemish-prone skin.[13]

Psychological Stress	Body's Response	Skin Effects
Acute	• Activates HPA axis, releasing stress hormones • Turns on adrenals (fight or flight response)	• Skin mast cells "turn on," promoting inflammation and skin sensitivity • Normal skin cell renewal cycles and activity are impaired
Chronic	• Surplus circulating steroid stress hormones, cortisol and catecholamines	• Increased circulating cortisol increases blood sugar levels, reducing insulin sensitivity and making skin more susceptible to advanced glycation end products (AGES) where sugar cross-links and breaks down healthy skin collagen and skin structure • Promotes sebum production, congesting skin and making it prone to blemishes and flare-ups • Disturbs and reduces skin microbiota diversity, increases "bad bacteria" overload, lowers skin pH and reduces barrier function, making skin more reactive to environmental assaults

Figure 1.1: The Impact of Emotional Stress on the Skin[14]

The gut-brain-skin axis is far more advanced and complicated than I have discussed here, but I hope you can see the impact and domino effect that our mental state can have on the health and appearance of the skin and skin microbiome, which you will learn more about in the next chapter. Research on the human microbiome continues to evolve and we are learning more and more about how probiotics can be used for mental health and cognition,

Good Bacteria for Healthy Skin

immunity, digestive health, weight management, skin health and more. As we learn more about the human microbiome, the ecosystem and activity of these microorganisms, this area of science will only become more practical within our own lives and perhaps over time will remap how we live and care for our well-being.

QUICK NUTRITION TIPS TO COMBAT STRESS (AND SAVE YOUR SKIN)

For most people, stress influences both the amount and types of food that they eat. Unfortunately, the food choices we make when we're stressed tend to be poor ones or "comfort foods," concentrated with sugar, trans fats, artificial fillers and preservatives.

It's hard to say no to those kinds of stress cravings, but nutrition should be a primary consideration for the management of stress. Because many nutrients are quickly depleted during the stress response, food choices should focus on supporting energy metabolism (physical and mental health), and hormonal and digestive health.

As we discuss the skin microbiome and the benefits of probiotics in the forthcoming chapters, I'll give more detailed recommendations and help you reveal healthy, luminous skin from the inside and out. But for now, here are some nutrition-focused suggestions to help "calm" and "de-stress" your mind and body.

Start by:

☀ Removing or limiting intake of sugar, caffeine and alcohol— all rob the body of essential nutrients (such as B vitamins), drain the adrenal glands, and fatigue the mind and body.

✳ Keeping meals simple and eating smaller meals more often, which is easier on the digestive system.

✳ Starting your day with a smoothie or opting for fresh juices (with no added sugar) in between meals. These provide concentrated doses of stress-busting nutrients to stabilize mood and energy.

✳ Don't forget about high-quality lean protein—proteins contain amino acids, essential for brain health and neurotransmitters.

Consume more:

✳ Seaweed and dark leafy greens—Nutrient-dense with vitamins and minerals including folate and magnesium (important in mood-regulating neurotransmitters, serotonin and dopamine). One of the easiest ways to get a green boost is adding them to your morning smoothies.

✳ Food with tryptophan, like turkey and eggs, and pumpkin seeds—Tryptophan is an amino acid needed to synthesize the neurotransmitter serotonin.

✳ Fermented foods—Stress strains the digestive system and gut microbiome. Probiotic foods such as fermented sauerkraut, kimchi, kombucha and pickled veggies encourage the growth of good bacteria in the gut. To help good bacteria flourish, choose prebiotic foods such as artichokes, garlic, beans, oats, onions and asparagus. Try to incorporate them more often in your diet, but start slowly so your digestive system can get used to them.

✳ Deep-colored berries (blueberries, blackberries, pomegranate)—These berries get their color from

anthocyanins, antioxidants that aid in the production of dopamine and combat oxidative stress in the body.

✳ Healthy-fat foods—High-fat cold water fish such as salmon, anchovies and sardines are rich in the omega-3 fatty acids eicosapentaenoic acid (EPA) and docosahexaenoic acid (DHA), which play an important role in our emotional well-being. Plant sources of omega-3 fatty acids include chia, hemp, walnuts, flax seeds and avocados (also good sources of magnesium). These fats also help to curb appetite and regulate blood sugar levels to keep energy and mood in balance.

✳ Adaptogenic herbs—These have been used traditionally for thousands of years in Eastern and European medicines. There are three criteria that classify an adaptogen: the ability to help the body resist stress help normalize bodily reactions during times of high stress, and have minimal side effects or toxicity. These plant-based compounds can help normalize and strengthen the body (adrenal glands, brain, heart, immune system) against the unfavorable effects of stress from the environment (physical, emotional, pollutants) on daily cellular reactions inside the body; adaptogens may counteract the degenerative effects of stress to support overall vitality.[15]

Some of the most commonly used adaptogens include ginseng, ashwagandha, rhodiola, amla (Indian gooseberry), cordyceps, holy basil, maca and more. Because some adaptogens work better for energy and vitality while others are best for their calming effects, it's important to do your research before considering an adaptogen and ensure there are no contraindications with your current health condition. Always consult a healthcare practitioner prior to use.

FIGURE 1.2: TOP NUTRIENTS TO COMBAT STRESS

STRESS NUTRIENT	WHY IT'S IMPORTANT	FOOD SOURCES
B Vitamins	These function as essential cofactors in the breakdown of carbohydrates to usable brain fuel and also support liver detoxification (if the liver is sluggish, hormones may become imbalanced). Also important in the production of the "feel good" neurotransmitter, serotonin.	Animal food sources, whole grains and bran, beans, peas, nuts. If following a vegan diet, supplement with B12 as it is mainly found in animal food sources.
Chromium (Cr) and Manganese (Mn)	Important minerals to balance blood sugar and insulin in the body. Chromium supports insulin, so glucose is properly balanced and utilized in the body. Manganese is required for the conversion of glucose to usable energy in the body.	Brewer's yeast, rye, oysters, potatoes, apples, bananas, spinach, molasses, chicken, seeds, beans, peas and leafy greens (if grown in organic, mineral-rich soil conditions).

STRESS NUTRIENT	WHY IT'S IMPORTANT	FOOD SOURCES
Fatty Acids	Combat deficiency in the brain associated with inflammation and interruption of normal function of nerve signaling. Two primary omega-3 fatty acids in the brain are DHA and EPA, which must be consumed regularly to maintain a constant supply in the brain. These fats also help to curb appetite and regulate blood sugar levels to keep energy and mood in balance.	Improve quality of all oil sources: Switch from refined and hydrogenated oils to unprocessed plant sources of essential fatty acids; choose whole grains (unmilled, freshly milled, sprouted); legumes and their sprouts; fresh nuts and seeds; dark green vegetables; and micro-algae. Use oils balanced in both linoleic and alpha-linolenic fatty acids such as flax seed, pumpkin seed and chia seed oils (note: use fresh oils cold pressed or refined). Consume EPA and DHA from fish, fish oils (salmon, sardine, anchovy) or spirulina.
Magnesium (Mg)	Essential for energy metabolism (conversion from food to usable energy) and promoting a calming effect on the body through the conversion and production of the relaxant hormone prostaglandin.	Green leafy vegetables, beans, peas, raw nuts and seeds, tofu, avocados, raisins, millet and other unrefined grains.
Potassium (K)	Essential for proper muscle and nerve function.	Abundant in raw fruits and vegetables, beans, peas, nuts and seeds.

STRESS NUTRIENT	WHY IT'S IMPORTANT	FOOD SOURCES
Vitamin C and Bioflavonoids	Some of the most important anti-stress and -fatigue nutrients, needed for health and hormone production of the adrenal glands. When under chronic stress, the adrenal glands become fatigued, increasing the need for vitamin C. Along with vitamin C, bioflavonoids offer antioxidant- and hormone-balancing properties to help even out mood and stress.	Citrus fruits (pulp and rind), peppers, grape skins, blackberries, blueberries. These nutrients cannot be stored in body, so it is important to replenish them daily.
Vitamin E	An important fat-soluble vitamin because it helps to relieve stress due to hormonal imbalance.	Best sources include avocado, wheat germ oil, walnuts and seed oils.
Zinc (Zn)	An important mineral to help calm mood by supporting proper blood sugar balance and digestion. Zinc helps with the digestion and action of the B vitamins and carbohydrate digestion.	Abundant in raw fruits and vegetables, beans, peas, nuts and seeds.

The Skin Microbiome—the Missing Link for Healthy Skin?

〜〜〜

In 2007 I started merging my experience in nutrition, medical aesthetics and nutraceuticals toward innovating and developing commercial dietary supplements for the skincare and personal care sectors. At that time there were very few beauty supplements on the market in North America. The few that were available had minimal research and lacked the consumer awareness seen in other places around the world. It was known as "nutricosmetics," or the concept that an integrative approach from diet, supplementation and topical care is essential for healthy skin and natural beauty. The concept of "beauty from within" was originally embraced in Asia and Europe. I remember walking into a pharmacy in Paris and

noticing many of the skincare brands offered some form of dietary supplement beside their skincare product. For me this was nothing new—I live by the idea that "you are what eat" and that over time this will reveal itself in your skin, outer appearance and how well you age. So why shouldn't you look at nutrition along with your topical regimens to reveal your own natural beauty? And why were we ignoring this concept in North America?

The early nutricosmetic formulations mostly focused on supportive antioxidant protection against environmental aggressors. Aggressors like UV exposure and urban pollution have been clinically proven to cause an influx of damaging reactive cells on the skin called "free radicals." Like a domino effect, free radicals rob healthy cells of an electron and in turn make them free radicals as well. Antioxidants can neutralize free radicals to stop them from damaging healthy skin cells. The free radical theory of aging is a leading factor in premature skin aging and mostly caused from the outside environment.

However, free radicals are not the only factors in premature skin aging. In 2015 and 2016, a second wave of nutricosmetics products gained mainstream attention in North America, this time focused around collagen. As we age, skin collagen production slows, as does skin metabolism. Wrinkles begin at the dermis, where the structural breakdown of skin collagen and elastin occurs (known as the skin collagen matrix). Today you see collagen-infused functional foods and supplements touting skin, hair and beauty benefits. The "collagen craze" in the last few years is what has accelerated consumer awareness and appreciation for the concept of "beauty from within."

More recently, the growing body of clinical evidence around the skin microbiome offers a third idea of how we may take better care for our skin. The concept of "balance" between bacteria groups and

their species is proposed to be a leading contributor to resilient, calm and moist skin. From where you live to what you consume, your personal hygiene and skincare practices can either harm or nurture your skin microbiome.

In essence, I see this as a trifold approach *from the inside and out* that includes three tiers for healthy skin and natural beauty:

1. Protect with antioxidants (through diet, supplementation, topical skincare, and SPF). I will discuss this in more detail in my microbiome plan in Chapters 7 and 8.

2. Strengthen with animal- or plant-based proteins, vitamins and minerals that are the building blocks for collagen production. Collagen peptides are an option to strengthen and firm skin connective tissue, hair and nails. I prefer marine or plant-based formulations over bovine, fowl or porcine.

3. Balance skin microflora with dietary, supplemental and topical care for calm, even, moist and balanced skin. This is where prebiotics and probiotics are influential; these will be discussed in upcoming chapters.

But first, to truly understand how diet and lifestyle can support and balance the skin microbiome, it's important to have a general idea of what makes for healthy skin.

STRUCTURE, FUNCTION AND IMPORTANCE OF THE SKIN MICROBIOME

Let's start with the basics. Bacteria's cell structure is simple, as they are single-cell microbes. They have no nucleus (the brains of the cell and the site of its DNA). Instead, bacteria contain its DNA

in a simple loop or structure. Bacteria are classified by their species type. Within one species, strains and subgroups can differ by where they live, how they survive, what disease they may produce and many other characteristics. They can also be distinguished by the nature of their cell walls, their shape or by differences in their genetic makeup. There are over 1 trillion different species of bacteria. Don't worry, there won't be a test! But it's important to understand just how complex bacteria can be, despite their relatively simple makeup.

You are the host to trillions of microbes that depend on you to survive, just as you depend on them for healthy, balanced skin. Microbes are introduced the instant you leave your mother's womb and evolve as you age. As an infant you are exposed to various environmental bacteria. As different areas of your skin develop moisture, temperature and glandular characteristics, distinctive skin microbial communities arise and become increasingly diverse over time. These microbial niches and their populations continue to change as you age, such as during puberty and with lifestyle and environmental exposure.[16]

As an adult your skin harbors a variety of bacterial communities that play a fundamental job in protecting you from your environment and supporting your skin immunity. We typically think of bacteria, fungi and viruses as harmful invaders, but in reality they can actually protect against pathogens, aggressors and toxins that can break down healthy skin.[17]

HOW SKIN MICROBES ARE TESTED

Scientists have been interested in microorganisms that inhabit the skin since Antonie van Leeuwenhoek, "the father of microbiology," made his first microscopic discoveries in 1674. In the 1950s, dermatology research

started using cell culture microbiology testing methods to identify microorganisms. Today, researchers are able to identify distinct species, their activity and their genetic footprint using 16S ribosomal RNA testing methods. The term "microbiome" was coined in 2001 by Nobel Laureate and geneticist Joshua Lederberg.[18] So even though the skin microbiome is a fairly new area of research, scientists have long questioned the nature of the relationship between humans and microorganisms. Today researchers are integrating their expertise to further understand and identify microorganisms that inhabit the skin and learn more about how their thriving ecosystem and diverse community is essential for healthy, balanced skin.

SKIN STRUCTURE

Your skin is the most extensive organ you have, weighing about 15 percent of your total body weight. Though it looks smooth and flat to the eye, it's composed of many grooves and three distinctive layers: the epidermis, dermis and hypodermis. One full skin cell cycle from the time a cell is produced to when it is pushed up to the outer epidermal layer and shed off your skin is about six weeks. However, skin cells renew on average every four weeks; this process slows with age.[19]

The epidermis (outermost layer) is the thinnest layer of skin and consists of keratin (a tough protein that reinforces the skin), Langerhans cells (which block foreign elements from getting into your skin) and melanocytes (which give skin its color). The epidermis also includes a skin layer called the "stratum corneum." This

is the very top non-living skin layer of the epidermis and main barrier from the external environment.

The dermis (middle layer) sits below the epidermis and is where wrinkles are first formed. The dermis contains blood vessels that nourish and oxygenate skin tissue, hair follicles and sebaceous (oil) glands. It is the site for new skin cell production and contains fibroblasts, cells that synthesize collagen and elastin, keeping skin smooth and firm.

The hypodermis (innermost layer) is what lies between the dermis and underlying tissues and organs. It consists of mostly loose connective and fat tissue, blood vessels and nerves that supply the skin, and serves to cushion us from impact and provide insulation. Your skin also contains different glands, including sebaceous glands (that produce sebum), eccrine glands (essential for temperature regulation and found throughout the skin) and apocrine glands (found in certain areas of the skin and the glands responsible for body odor).[20]

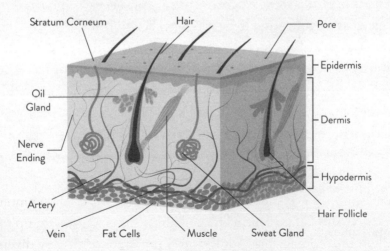

Now take a look at your face in the mirror or glance at your arms and legs. What you see are your keratinocytes, those protein-packed

cells that make up most of the epidermis. As noted, the epidermis is a tough physical barrier that resists entry from harmful pathogens and toxins while retaining moisture and nutrients inside the body.[21] That outermost layer, the stratum corneum, is a collection of a unique type of keratinocytes called squames. These are flattened cells packed with protein-rich keratin cross-linked and embedded in fat (lipid bilayers) to form the "brick and mortar" of the epidermis. This is also where skin microflora is most active, but studies show bacteria also reside within the deeper layers of the epidermis and into the living skin tissue below.[22]

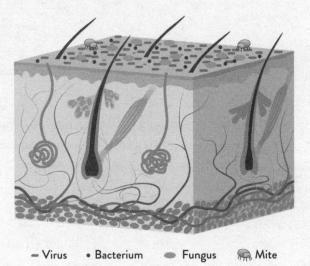

— Virus   • Bacterium   ⬭ Fungus   🕷 Mite

WHAT CONSTITUTES A HEALTHY SKIN MICROBIOTA?

Your skin is a complex ecosystem of diverse bacterial communities. A single square centimeter of human skin can contain up to 1 billion microorganisms. Adult skin is inhabited by highly diverse communities of bacterial populations.[23] Your skin microbiome is also unique to you based on your genotype, age, sex, diet, hygiene,

lifestyle and the environment you live in. These trillions of bacteria, fungi and viruses that live on our skin make up the skin microbiome.[24]

The skin microbiota (or skin flora) includes two groups:

1. Resident microorganisms (the hosts) that are routinely found on the skin, which adapt and reestablish themselves in changing environments. These microorganisms are usually harmless and provide some benefit to the skin.

2. Transient microorganisms (the tourists), which do not establish permanent residency on the skin but arise from environmental exposure and last for hours or days before vanishing. Typically, "the tourists" are also non-pathogenic.[25]

These bacteria can form mutualistic (where both host and microbe benefit), commensal (where one benefits) or detrimental (where host and/or microbe are harmed) relationships with our skin. It is our skin's immune system that acts to manage the microbial communities and maintain beneficial microbe-host relationships.[26]

Your skin provides different environments for bacteria to reside on as well. Dry versus humid regions of the body typically determine the type of bacterial communities that reside and evolve there. Your skin has three major ecologic environments: dry (e.g., forearm, buttocks, back), moist (e.g., underarm, inner elbow, groin) and sebaceous (e.g., scalp). Bacterial diversity seems to be greatest on dry skin environments. Although there are general characteristics for the human skin microbiome, both the composition and the abundance of skin microbes vary between us and continually evolve and adapt based on our age, health and the environment we are exposed to. As adults, there are generally four major phyla or groups of bacteria on our skin areas: Actinobacteria,

Proteobacteria, Firmicutes and Bacteroidetes.[27] Within those phyla, Staphylococcus, Corynebacterium and Propionibacterium account for over 60 percent of the bacterial types present on the skin. Bacteria can also obtain their nourishment from the sebum, sweat and fats on our skin.[28]

THE KEY PLAYERS

Our skin is actually an undesirable environment for bacteria; it is acidic, low in moisture, covered in salt-laden sweat and full of antibacterial molecules. Additionally, it is constantly exposed to pollutants and aggressors from our outside environment.[29] Notwithstanding this, bacteria have found a way not only to live but also thrive on and become normal flora within the skin.[30] This balance is called a state of symbiosis.

There are three key bacterial types (genera) that have adapted well to life on our skin and dominate over other microbes.

Staphylococcus is a type of bacteria containing at least 28 species, also known jointly as Staphylococci. Although there are some species that can cause infectious diseases, most of them do not. *S. epidermidis* is the most predominant skin strain (subspecies), but many others including *S. hominis*, *S. capitis* and *S. saprophyticus* are also present. When viewed under a microscope they appear circular and when clumped together resemble a bunch of grapes. As they have the ability to survive with or without oxygen, they are most prevalent on the skin but prefer moister areas. They can withstand high salt content in sweat. While they can be responsible for sweat odor, they are important in strengthening the skin barrier and releasing additional nutrients for the skin. *S. epidermidis* also has the ability to create an enzyme to slow the growth

of and protect against certain harmful bacteria such as *S. aureus*, bacteria that can cause invasive skin infections and/or toxin-type conditions, including food poisoning and toxic shock syndrome. The overuse of topical and oral antibiotics can be damaging to this group of healthy skin bacteria.[31]

Corynebacterium are a group of bacteria most predominantly found on moist and sebaceous skin sites and include *C. accolens*, *C. jeikeium*, *C. urealyticum*, *C. amycolatum*, *C. minutissimum* and *C. striatum*. Corynebacterium are "lipid-loving" bacteria and must obtain fats from their environment; thus, they thrive on oilier areas of the skin. They can also flourish in a high-salt environment and may rely on some of the vitamins in sweat for survival. Certain strains have been implicated in chronic skin conditions including erythrasma (a condition causing brown patches, and itchy, scaly skin) and pitted keratolysis (a bacterial infection found on soles of feet and palms.)[32]

Propionibacterium is an anaerobic bacterium found in low-oxygen environments on the skin, in pores and on hair follicles, where it feeds on sebaceous matter (the fatty substance produced in glands to keep skin waterproof). *P. acnes*, also known commonly as simply acne, is the best-known member, but several others are found regularly on skin, such as *P. avidum* and *P. granulosum*. Through its presence in pores and follicles, it can help the skin by stopping harmful bacteria from getting into the pores. *P. acnes* also produces arginine, an amino acid and energy source for skin proteins. This bacterium increases enormously during puberty and produces compounds that can put skin out of balance, producing blemishes. When in balance, this bacterium builds a strong barrier against foreign invaders; however, the overuse of antibacterial soaps can destroy its natural ecosystem and balance.[33]

When you think of how these and other bacteria work as a living ecosystem alongside our skin, how can they contribute to its overall health? Scientists are learning more each day and propose the following ways our microbiome helps our skin:

1. Protects us. Our "home" or resident skin bacteria create a barrier or biofilm that provides the first line of defense against harmful pathogens and aggressors. Certain resident strains can also inhibit the growth and activity of harmful bacteria.

2. Supports and strengthens skin immunity. Your skin is a powerful immune organ that has a synergistic relationship with the microbiome, and they are in constant communication. Some bacterial strains have the ability to "turn up" the skin's immune response, and others help to minimize inflammation after skin has been wounded or injured.

3. Boosts skin barrier function. Skin flora interact and potentially influence the physical skin barrier that helps protect us from environmental aggressors and lock in skin moisture. *Staphylococcus aureus* and Corynebacterium in general have been shown to produce byproducts or stimulate reactions that promote skin's natural moisturizing factor.[34]

AVOIDING DYSBIOSIS

When the skin's equilibrium is disrupted, it is in a state of dysbiosis. This is what we're trying to avoid. Changes in the activity and composition of skin bacteria or an immune response can trigger inflammation, accelerated skin aging and other chronic conditions that I will highlight now and discuss in more detail in later chapters.[35]

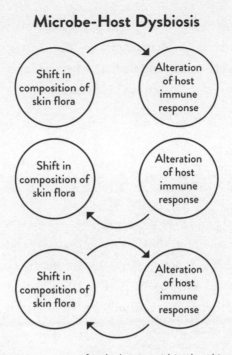

Microbe-Host Dysbiosis

Shift in composition of skin flora

Alteration of host immune response

Shift in composition of skin flora

Alteration of host immune response

Shift in composition of skin flora

Alteration of host immune response

Figure 2.1. Dysbiosis is a state of imbalance within the skin microbiota that negatively affects the host. This shift in skin microbiota can be influenced by different lifestyle and environmental factors that alter the skin flora composition and potentially suppress skin immunity and encourage chronic inflammation.

DYSBIOSIS AND YOUR SKIN MICROBIOME

As a living ecosystem, your skin microbiome is constantly adapting and in communication with you. When it is balanced, this is called a state of "symbiosis." But when there is an imbalance with the microbiota, it's a state of "dysbiosis." Dysbiosis can be caused by our environment or products we apply to our skin that alter the composition of its microflora. It can also be triggered by our nutrition and health status, which affect our immunity and/or promote systemic inflammation. In either case, these interferences upset the normal balance of the microbiota and are believed to contribute to skin inflammation and certain diseases.[36]

Good Bacteria for Healthy Skin

ATOPIC DERMATITIS

Atopic dermatitis is a condition that makes the skin red, uncomfortable and itchy. It is common in children but can affect any age. Research on the skin microbiome has found that people with this condition tend to have an overload of harmful bacteria *S. aureus* on the affected skin sites.[37] The overcolonization of *S. aureus* is thought to negatively impact skin's natural balance and microbial diversity, and increases the likelihood of this particular skin condition. Other studies have found that fungus and other potentially harmful bacteria can also aggravate skin immunity, making skin hypersensitive and increasing the risk of atopic dermatitis. Studies have also found a correlation between gut microflora diversity and imbalance with atopic dermatitis.[38]

PSORIASIS

Psoriasis is a chronic autoimmune condition that triggers a rapid accumulation of skin cells. It creates itchy red skin with a silvery scaled appearance and is more commonly found on the elbows, knees and scalp. Although psoriasis is generally considered a genetic condition, microorganisms have been connected to it since the 1950s, when it was thought that psoriasis was related to the bacteria that causes throat infections.[39] More recently, research has found that an overabundance of certain bacterial strains, namely strains within the Proteobacterium and Streptococcus groups, are more active in psoriasis than in healthy skin, affecting the diversity of the skin microbiota.[40] Another study was able to identify that psoriasis patients had less microbial diversity than those with healthy skin.[41] Although there are other factors to consider with psoriasis, what is interesting to note is the lack of microbial diversity associated with skin sites affected by the psoriasis condition.[42]

ACNE VULGARIS

From blackheads and whiteheads to pimples, "acne vulgaris" is a technical term for what we commonly know as "acne." We have all experienced a breakout at one point in our lives, but when it becomes chronic and severe, it can also cause long-lasting and unsightly scarring. The condition involves a blockage and/or inflammation of the hair follicles and the sebaceous glands that surround them, which causes a blemish. Although there is a hybrid of factors associated with acne vulgaris, the involvement of microbes is one of the main causes. *Propionibacterium acnes* is the dominant microorganism that colonizes and takes over skin microflora within those blemish-prone areas. This dysbiosis is coupled with inflammation, and the overproduction of sebum exacerbates this condition.[43] One study also identified that these pathogenic strains have the ability to become antibiotic-resistant, which means an integrative approach is best for managing this acne.[44]

DANDRUFF

Dandruff is a condition affecting the scalp that causes skin flaking and itching. To date, it is mostly treated with antifungal-type products, but more recent research indicates that an imbalance in scalp microflora may also be a key factor in dandruff. One study looking at the physiological conditions associated with this condition found that bacteria, rather than fungi, was the strongest predictor that determined the severity of dandruff. For future treatments, researchers suggested that products work to rebalance scalp microflora to better manage and support a healthy scalp.[45]

SENSITIVE SKIN

Sensitive skin is a condition that can involve skin tightness, stinging, burning, tingling and redness in response to factors that normally shouldn't provoke this type of reaction. Although the research is still in early stages, there is a suggestion that impaired stratum corneum (that outer visible layer of skin and site where microbes are most active) and changes in skin's pH create dysbiosis. These combined effects may be a cause of hyperreactive or sensitive skin.[46]

CHAPTER 3

Lifestyle and the Skin Microbiome

~~~

In 2005, the American cancer epidemiologist Christopher Wild created the term "exposome" to describe the totality of exposures that an individual experiences throughout their life.[47] As one of the two organs visible to the outside environment (the eyes being the other), our skin is under lifelong exposure to an array of stressors. In 2016, European scientists collaborated to define and identify what they called the "skin aging exposome." Their work brought forth a definition of the skin aging exposome along with the hybrid of contributing factors that accelerate skin aging.[48]

Factors affecting the skin aging exposome fall into the following major categories:

* Sun and digital radiation

* Air pollution, smog

* Tobacco smoke

* Nutrition

* Stress and lack of sleep

* Cosmetic products[49]

Today, research in skin aging is moving beyond "sun protection factor" (SPF) and toward a more integrated "life protection factor," which focuses on how our environment (sun rays, digital rays and pollution), lifestyle, diet and mental health influence the health, aging and appearance of our skin.[50] Since the skin microbiome is most active on our exposed skin, it only makes sense to narrow our view on some of these elements included in the skin aging exposome and look at their potential effect on the skin microbiome.

WE ALL EMIT A "BIOME CLOUD"

Our skin microbiome is highly adaptable and varies widely among individuals in comparison to the gut microbiome. This "biome cloud" is influenced not only by our age, genetics and health status but also by our environment, lifestyle, pets, foods we consume and products we apply on our skin. Interestingly, people who reside in rural settings and are in daily contact with nature are exposed to more diverse microorganisms that help diversify skin microflora and strengthen immunity.[51] It is believed that being surrounded by microbe-rich soil allows the skin to be in contact with a variety of microbes that can strengthen the skin ecosystem and control the spread of potentially harmful pathogens on the skin.[52]

On the flip side, as urbanization continues to demolish green space and expand cities, we are less exposed to naturally occurring microorganisms that have nurtured our adaptability and strength against disease.[53] A lack of biodiversity in the gut and

skin microbiomes[51] has been connected to the increase in autoimmune, inflammatory, skin and mental health conditions.[54] Modern lifestyles and urbanization are challenging researchers to rethink the widely recognized "hygiene hypothesis" and turn their attention to the "biodiversity hypothesis," which suggests that reduced exposure to natural microbial communities increases risk of autoimmune diseases.[55] As the research proves, there is such a thing as being "too clean," despite what our mothers might have said when we were kids!

> As highlighted in a World Allergy Organization Consensus Statement, "biodiversity loss leads to reduced interaction between environmental and human microbiotas. This in turn may lead to immune dysfunction and impaired tolerance mechanisms in humans."[56]

THE STRATUM CORNEUM AND SKIN MICROBIOME WORKING TOGETHER

Think about what your skin is exposed to from the air and environment. From synthetics in our clothing to chemicals in our skincare, it is amazing how resilient our skin can be. Our skin provides us with a first line of defense, protecting both passively and dynamically through different mechanisms.[57] We often refer to our skin as a "barrier" from our external environment, but it works more like a filter, allowing some diffusion of environmental microbes, chemicals and byproducts to penetrate into the deeper layers of the skin and potentially reach the bloodstream. If you recall, the outer visible layer of skin, the stratum corneum, is where the skin microbiome is most active. The stratum corneum and microbiome

work closely together in regulating what penetrates the skin. This constant interaction between the stratum corneum, skin microbiome and the environment can have a significant influence on our skin and total immune networks.[58] When the stratum corneum and microbiome are healthy and balanced, our immune defense and ability to ward off aggressors and environmental stressors is resilient. You can see in the chart below the many factors your skin microbiome interacts with every day.

FIGURE 3.1: RELATIONSHIP OF MICROBES BETWEEN HUMANS (HOST), ANIMALS AND THE ENVIRONMENT

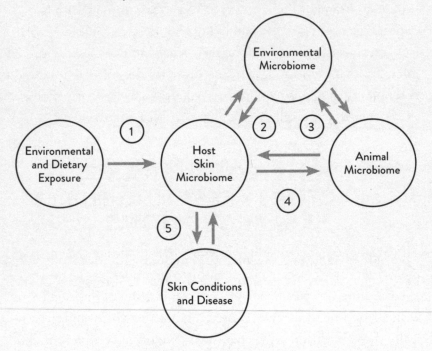

1. Pollution, diet, topicals and antibiotic exposure—Antibiotics and medications, shifts in diet, cosmetics/skincare, air pollutants and UV rays can alter the diversity and stability of the skin and human microbiomes.

2. Environment—Urbanization and indoor environments can hinder exposure to the microbes essential for healthy skin and human microbiomes.

3 and 4. Environment/pets and host—Cohabitation with animals helps diversify (and strengthen) the skin microbiome. This has been shown in studies with children and the reduced incidence of allergies in those who have pets.

5. Skin microbiome's influence on conditions/disease—These environmental and lifestyle exposures influence the health of the skin microbiome, which in turn has an effect on the health and appearance of the skin. Urban living and lifestyle combined with lack of exposure to nature and green space limits contact with microbes that help strengthen and diversify the skin microbiome and immunity against conditions including sensitive or reactive skin, acne, atopic dermatitis, eczema, rosacea and dandruff.[59]

ENVIRONMENTAL FACTORS AFFECTING THE SKIN MICROBIOME

There are several ways in which the environment affects our skin. In this chapter we'll talk about the top two: UV/digital rays and pollution.

UV AND DIGITAL RAYS

Our skin is constantly under stress from ultraviolet rays, pollution and chemical byproducts we apply on our skin. Along with sun exposure, clinical evidence also suggests that our constant interaction with digital rays from computers and mobile phones exposes our skin to oxidative stressors that play a central role in premature

skin aging.[60] Our constant interaction with this radiation has been shown to change our natural skin biology; researchers refer to this as "toasted skin syndrome." Devices like tablets, smartphones and laptops can also intensify UV reflection. One study found that in comparison to people not using cell phones or tablets, UV reflections increased by 36 percent with cell phones and up to 85 percent when using tablets such as iPads.[61]

So how does this affect the skin microbiome? One of the major effects of UV rays on microbes is DNA damage, which can change the livelihood and activity of the microbial communities that normally reside on the skin.[62] UV rays also suppress the immune system. Skin microbes and the immune system are in constant communication to maintain equilibrium. When skin microbes are weakened, infectious pathogens can more easily invade the skin.[63] Chronic exposure to UV rays leads to a change in quantity, activity and spread of the health-promoting microorganisms, and by upsetting the normal functioning between the immune system and resident microbial communities, your skin becomes more sensitive and potentially susceptible to harmful pathogens and invaders.[64]

POLLUTION

Environmental scientists have started to look at the potential connection between increased air pollution and the skin, such as in the rise of adult acne. Recent studies have shown that chronic high exposure to air pollutants have been associated with premature skin aging and inflammatory or allergic skin conditions.[65] This is because your skin acts as a "sponge" for certain chemical air pollutants, such as polycyclic aromatic hydrocarbons (PAHs), volatile organic compounds (VOCs), oxides, particulate matter (PM), ozone (O_3) and cigarette smoke.[66] These toxins build up in skin,

clogging pores, depleting oxygen to cells and breaking down skin structure and function.

To look at the relationship between pollution and its potential effect on the skin microbiome, researchers in China took 231 female volunteers who live in large cities (with a population over 1 million) and megacities (with a population over 10 million). They assessed the gene activity of microorganisms taken from cheek swabs from both groups. The study found that there were well-defined differences in the skin microbiomes of women living in the megacities versus those in large cities. The most noticeable difference was variation in the composition of the biome—there was less microbial diversity for the women living in the megacities. The researchers also noticed that those women living in megacities had a more fragile microbial network because of the lower microbial diversity and density, making the skin more reactive and sensitive to chronic conditions. They concluded that the higher rate of skin diseases in megacities is largely due to a less robust skin microbiome.[67]

It isn't surprising to learn that pollution has a negative impact on the health of our skin. What is interesting to learn is *how* it impacts the skin. Based on the current evidence, there are different routes of action:

❋ Air pollutants, such as carbon monoxide, heavy metals, nitrogen oxides, ozone, sulfur dioxide, volatile organic vapors and particulate matters, can induce oxidative stress in resident skin microbes, leading to a microbiome collapse and making skin more susceptible to damage.[68]

❋ Exposed skin is composed of skin cells rich in lipids and proteins that can become damaged when exposed to urban pollutants. Skin antioxidant content also becomes depleted,

weakening the skin barrier and allowing the potential for toxins to reach the deeper layers of skin. Pollutants can then induce a flow of inflammatory reactions that offset the normal functioning of skin cells.[69]

❋ Since the skin microbiome resides mostly on the stratum corneum, normal residual skin microbes are also upset from air pollution. One study observed a 50 percent decrease in residual skin microflora in the presence of ozone.[70] Alterations in microbe diversity and overactivity of pathogenic strains of bacteria such as *Propionibacterium acnes* (the main strain responsible for acne) have been confirmed in studies on exposed polluted skin.[71]

❋ Pollution particles settle on the skin, clogging pores and limiting oxygenation to the tissue. This causes a shift in skin pH and sebum production, along with a decrease in skin antioxidants like vitamin E, making a perfect environment for inflammatory and bacterial skin conditions.[72]

CHALLENGING THE "HYGIENE HYPOTHESIS"

As a society we are obsessed with cleaning products! From sterilizing agents to antibacterial soaps and disinfectants, our constant scrubbing and cleaning products are having a negative effect on our skin microbiome.

Our overreliance on disinfecting could be providing new opportunities for resistant and potentially harmful pathogens to invade our skin.[73] Remember that the microbiome is a dynamic and colonized community of microorganisms that work closely with the immune system to maintain a state of symbiosis. If we are

continually exposing our skin to antimicrobials and antibiotics that strip away offending pathogens along with health-promoting "resident" colonizing communities, how can the skin maintain a state of symbiosis? The answer is it cannot.

Yet our hands are the gateway for most germ transmission and a common cause of outbreaks in clinical and hospital settings. Clinically validated antimicrobial soaps that remove bacteria and viruses usually contain ethanol, isopropanol or n-propanol. These products have been shown to remove bacteria and viruses by up to 80 percent.[74] Soap and water is the other preferred method in clinical settings.[75]

SEVEN STEPS TO WASH YOUR HANDS PROPERLY

Hands are the main pathways of germ transmission in healthcare. The World Health Organization recommends a seven-step hand washing protocol to avoid the transmission of harmful germs and prevent healthcare-associated infections. The whole process should take 20 to 60 seconds depending on how dirty your hands are. Alcohol-based cleansers or soap and water are preferred. These can be a good alternative when you don't have access to soap and water. Look for a product that contains at least 60% alcohol.

Step 1—Wet your hands and apply enough soap (coin size).

Step 2—Rub your palms together.

Step 3—Rub the back of each hand.

Step 4—Rub both your hands while interlocking your fingers.

Step 5—Rub the backs of your fingers.

Step 6—Rub the tips of your fingers.

Step 7—Rub your thumbs and your wrists.[76]

With proper hand washing, we can reduce the spread and contamination of germs. But it is the constant overuse and reliance on disinfectants that may be tipping the natural ecology of our skin, making it more vulnerable to harmful microbes and the environment. In addition, your skin is slightly acidic, at or slightly below a pH of 5 (and those healthy microbes thrive in a slightly acidic state).[77] Soap, however, is alkaline at a pH of 10! One study found that skin microflora thrived best and clung to skin at a pH of 4 to 4.5 while a more alkaline pH of 8 to 9 caused a scattering of those healthy microbes.[78] So with our overuse of sanitizers, we are in fact weakening our skin microbiome.

Hand sanitizers, topical and internal medications can also *harm* the skin microbiome. Think of it this way: To fight the spread of an infection, topical antibiotics and antiseptics are used to restrain the colonization of more pathogenic bacteria. But how do antibiotics and antiseptic agents effect the total microbial communities? They wipe out everything! Our overreliance on soaps and disinfectants, as well as chronic use of antibiotic medications, is also wiping out the good microbes and colonies that keep your skin healthy. One animal study found that skin treated with antibiotics caused an immediate shift in bacterial residents and stayed this way several days after treatment.[79] Antiseptics were not as strong in their effect but also caused minor changes in the skin bacterial populations. Both antibiotics and antiseptics decreased the growth and activity of Staphylococcus, a major resident group of bacteria that competes and controls the potentially harmful growth of *S. aureus* pathogen. Researchers then retreated the skin

with the healthy bacterial strain of Staphylococcus (that were previously disrupted by antibiotic and antiseptics), and found that the ability to fight off *S. aureus* was reduced by over 100-fold! They concluded that although antibiotics and antiseptics work to fight the spread of bacterial infection, they also negatively impact the viability and balance of resident skin microflora that protect the skin from potentially harmful pathogens.[80]

Another study looked at the effects of the two most common orally prescribed antibiotics—amoxicillin and azithromycin—and whether short-term use has a long-term effect on human microbiota. They sampled feces, saliva and skin specimens over six months from a group of people living together. They found a significant change in microbiota diversity in the gut and mouth with some effect on skin in as little as three days of oral antibiotic use. Those who took amoxicillin for seven days had the greatest shift and reduction in microbial diversity. The study concluded that commonly prescribed antibiotics can result in sustained reductions in microbiota diversity, which could have implications for the maintenance of human health and resilience to disease.[81] Although antibiotics are a core treatment for acute bacterial infections worldwide, our overreliance on them is potentially diminishing our natural ability to protect ourselves against harmful pathogens over the long term.

With these and more recent studies suggesting that microbes are essential for maintaining skin health, it is becoming clear that it may be time to challenge the rationale that hygiene products must remove all microbes. Rather, products should aim to diminish pathogenic organisms and simultaneously increase or maintain those resident microorganisms that help protect skin and maintain symbiosis.[82] Through advanced testing methods and research, scientists continue to discover new gene identities and activities

of specific bacterial strains that will help to leverage these types of products now and into the future.[83] We will dive into this in more detail in Chapters 5 and 7 on probiotics for skincare.

TOPICALS AND COSMETICS

By definition, a personal care product is a non-medicinal product that is intended for topical care and the grooming of the body and hair without affecting the structure or functions of the body. They are used for cleansing, toning, moisturizing, hydrating, exfoliating, conditioning, smoothing, soothing, deodorizing, perfuming and styling.[84]

And we love our products! When I walk into a beauty store, I'm often overwhelmed by the enormous number of products available for our skin and hair. Once upon a time, a three-step process—cleanse, moisturize and apply SPF—was all that was recommended for healthy skin. Today, multiple steps with many products and gadgets are advertised to help you achieve a glow. Then you apply makeup, including foundation, BB creams, eye shadows, blush, highlighters, powders...can you imagine how many chemicals you apply to your skin each day? According to a survey conducted on 2,300 people by the Environmental Working Group, the average adult uses nine personal care products each day, with 126 unique chemical ingredients.[85] Some of these ingredients have been highlighted in research and media for their potential health concerns, and this is one of the reasons why the Environmental Working Group created a Cosmetics Database that highlights commonly used personal care ingredients, what they're used for and their overall safety profile.[86]

Topical creams, powders, lotions, sprays and other cosmetics contain chemicals and preservatives that can alter the skin microbiome.[87]

In preliminary studies, it is suggested that the preservatives used to maintain shelf life of topical products can reduce the diversity and decrease the number of resident microbes. And as you know by now, this change in colonization and composition of the skin microflora can cause a shift in how the microbiome adapts and defends itself from the environment.[88] What is exciting to know is that the emerging cultural shift and demand for natural, non-synthetic skincare is advancing formulation and manufacturing technologies to produce more stable, more effective and less abrasive products for the market. The evolution of advocate groups and increasing number of "clean beauty" brands offers a platform for transparency and education to look beyond the package and truly understand those ingredients printed on a label. Clean eating and clean beauty are growing synonymously with superfoods and plant-based ingredients are becoming more mainstream. This is also true for pre- and probiotics and their unique benefits for health and beauty as they relate to our microbiome. We will learn more about this in Chapter 5.

THE DIRTY DOZEN

Although we're hearing more about clean beauty these days, it isn't a new topic, but rather a growing area of concern as we become more aware of the health effects of chemicals used in cosmetics. In 2010, the environmental advocate group David Suzuki Foundation published a report called the "Dirty Dozen, Cosmetic Chemicals to Avoid." They reported that one in eight ingredients used in personal care products is an industrial chemical, including carcinogens, pesticides, reproductive toxins and hormone disruptors. Many products include plasticizers (chemicals that keep concrete soft), degreasers

(used to get grime off auto parts) and surfactants (reduce surface tension in water, like in paint and inks).

The report highlighted the following ingredients as the "Dirty Dozen" to be aware of:

1. BHA and BHT
2. Coal tar and dyes
3. DEA
4. Dibutyl phthalate
5. Formaldehyde-releasing preservatives
6. Parabens
7. Parfum (aka fragrance)
8. PEG compounds
9. Petrolatum
10. Siloxanes
11. Sodium laureth sulfate
12. Triclosan[89]

DIET

As mentioned in Chapter 1, your gut microbiome is connected to your skin microbiome. This gut-skin axis has been linked with several skin conditions such as acne vulgaris, atopic dermatitis and psoriasis.[90] Inflammation and barrier defects or "leaky gut" (when undigested byproducts and toxins enter the bloodstream) also have an influence on the health of your skin. For example, gut bacterial overgrowth or dysbiosis has been found to increase the risk of acne.[91] Since digestion is the gateway to how we absorb and metabolize energy and nutrients and excrete toxins, why wouldn't you consider nutrition a fundamental component for healthy skin? Interestingly, this is not a new area of investigation; in fact, in 1911, a gastroenterologist named Milton H. Mack recommended that science look to the gut as an influence on skin conditions such as acne and eczema.[92]

The modern Western diet has been implicated in many chronic diseases because it lacks nutrient density and relies on chemically

laden foods that offer little or no nutrition value. Like a domino effect, what we consume directly affects our gut health, which then impacts our skin. Here's how:

❋ Our diet exposes us to microbes that have the ability to change gut microflora and signaling byproducts that reach and communicate with the skin.

❋ Those signaling byproducts derived from the gut have the ability to alter the diversity and activity of skin microflora.

❋ Chemicals and toxins we ingest through diet can bypass the gut and enter the bloodstream, affecting the skin microbiome.[93]

We can't ignore the influence of diet and the close relationship between the gut and skin. Many factors go into the connection, but what we consume does have an indirect effect on the ecology and health of the skin microbiome. From foods to oral probiotic strains that can effectively manage inflammatory skin conditions such as acne, the gut helps to regulate skin immune function and impacts the natural ecology of the skin microflora.[94]

In this chapter we learned about how the microbiome adapts to or is changed by what we expose it to. We also learned that what we have typically thought of as "good" may in fact be harming the natural stability and strength of the skin microbiome. As a living ecosystem, your skin microbiome wraps itself around you, interacting with and adapting to your external environment while helping to protect you from harmful invaders. If we do not care for it in such a way that healthy microbes can thrive and flourish, we may increase our risk of certain skin conditions. This is what we'll move onto in Chapter 4.

Skin Conditions Associated with the Skin Microbiome

〜〜〜

This new understanding of the skin microbiome as a dynamic and living ecosystem as discussed in previous chapters is shifting our approach in how we care for our skin. It is encouraging the innovation of integrative approaches and products to protect, nourish and balance the skin microbiome.

The focus for this chapter is to discuss in more detail conditions affected by the skin microbiome, along with providing an introduction to pre- and probiotics and their relative importance to restore and balance the skin from the inside and out.

INTRODUCTION TO PROBIOTICS AND PREBIOTICS

I'm sure if you're reading this book, you're already familiar with or have heard about probiotics and possibly prebiotics. Their evolving health benefits continue to be illuminated as research on the human microbiome advances. We see them marketed on food labels, dietary supplements and, more recently, in skincare products. But what exactly are they and how are they relevant to healthy skin?

With the growing acceptance that the human microbiome is a significant factor in our health, finding ways to support it has put probiotics in the spotlight. Probiotics are living microbes that, when consumed as a food or dietary supplement, have a beneficial effect on you (the host). They have been extensively studied on infants to adults for their benefits for gastrointestinal health and immunity, and for their influence on cognitive and skin health (the gut-brain-skin axis theory).[95]

Most probiotics fall into the group of lactic acid–producing bacteria normally consumed from foods such as yogurt and fermented milks. In food manufacturing, probiotics provide antimicrobial properties, enhance flavors and/or improve the nutritional value or bioavailability of nutrients. Probiotics offer a large scope of health benefits, including:

✺ Stabilizing intestinal health by balancing pH, promoting healthy gut microflora, detoxifying/neutralizing harmful pathogens, and improving absorption and bioavailability of nutrients from diet and supplementation.

✺ Strengthening and balancing the immune system to help manage inflammation and allergic responses in the body.[96]

Good Bacteria for Healthy Skin

While their popularity has grown recently, probiotics have been around for a long time. They were used traditionally to ferment foods and extend shelf life. Foods naturally containing probiotics include acidophilus milk/yogurt, cottage cheese, cultured butter and buttermilk, kefir, kimchi, kombucha tea, miso, pickles, sauerkraut and soy sauce.[97]

Since the typical Western diet is filled with processed and chemically preserved foods, we consume fewer probiotic-rich foods today than our ancestors did. Conventional farming and manufacturing methods also diminished nutrient density in our food, subsequently promoting a state of chronic low-grade inflammation in the body. This continuing state of systemic inflammation stresses our bodies and is thought to be a precursor to many chronic conditions or diseases, including those of the skin.[98] With probiotics' influence on regulating immune and inflammatory responses, they offer a promising option for balancing skin health through the microbiome and immune system. I could write a book on probiotics alone because the health benefits are that vast! But our interest here is to understand their innate connection and effect on the skin microbiome.[99]

PROBIOTICS

Probiotics are internationally recognized as live microorganisms that, when administered in adequate amounts, offer a health benefit to the host.[100] They are named and recognized according to their group (genus) species and subspecies, if applicable. So, you may see a probiotic listed as "*Lactobacillus plantarum* HY7714," where "Lactobacillus" is the genus, "plantarum" is the species and HY7714 is the specific strain/subspecies.

A probiotic must have the ability to:

1. Exert a beneficial effect on the host;

2. Remain active and viable throughout the shelf life of the product;

3. Survive transit through the GI tract, adhere to the intestinal lining and colonize in the tract;

4. Produce antimicrobial substances toward pathogens; and

5. Stabilize the intestinal microflora and be associated with health benefits.

The most extensively studied and widely used probiotics are the lactic acid bacteria, particularly the Lactobacillus and Bifidobacterium species.[101]

Note: Processing and heating can destroy probiotics, so look for labels that say, "Contains live and active cultures."

PREBIOTICS

Though probiotics and prebiotics sound alike, they are different from each other and offer different health benefits. Probiotics are live, beneficial bacteria naturally created through the process of fermentation. Prebiotics are a type of dietary fiber found in fruits, vegetables and legumes. When consumed through diet, prebiotics provide a source of fuel for microbes already present in the gut and colon. They also stimulate the growth and activity of good bacteria to improve the health and balance of the gut microbiome.[102] Prebiotics are not affected by stomach acid or heat processing, making them more stable than probiotics, but we should consume them more often to attain their health benefits (recommendations indicate we should get about 5 grams of prebiotic fiber per day versus the 2 to 3 grams generally consumed in the modern diet).[103] The most common prebiotics are inulin and oligofructose, both

found in plant-based foods. By increasing your intake of fiber, you will also boost your intake of prebiotics, but take note of the most nutrient-dense sources, which include chicory root, onions and garlic, oats, asparagus, dandelion greens, barley, apple skins, Jerusalem artichokes, bananas, leeks, flaxseeds, wheat bran and seaweed.[104]

MICROBES, PRE- AND PROBIOTICS, AND CHRONIC SKIN CONDITIONS

The skin is a complex network of interactions between microbes, epidermal cells and immune receptors. When an imbalance of microorganisms occurs, it can affect how the immune system responds to environmental aggressors or products applied to the skin. It can also affect the overall health and function of skin tissue. This is where pre- and probiotics can be helpful. With the growing body of promising clinical evidence, pre- and probiotics could provide options to help normalize the skin's ecosystem and manage chronic skin conditions.[105]

ACNE VULGARIS

Acne is brought on by a number of different factors including inflammation, oxidative stress, fluctuating hormones and insulin levels, and excess sebum and keratin production within the hair follicle on the skin. Whiteheads (or comedones) develop in the hair follicles where they become dilated and congested with skin debris, bacteria and sebum. Over the years, acne has become more common in adulthood. Experts cite external factors including diet, lifestyle, stress and pollution as drivers in its progression. Because of the multiple influences that contribute to acne, the "acne exposome" was created from consensus meetings in 2017 by European

dermatologists. It is based on the sum of contributing categories that are associated with acne, including nutrition, medication and occupational factors such as cosmetics, pollutants, climate, psychology and lifestyle.[106]

In earlier chapters, we learned that the skin microbiome is also associated with acne. The balance and mixture of skin microbes can influence the onset and severity of acne or blemish-prone skin.[107] Acne-prone skin has less microbial diversity and balance between two normally present residential bacteria: *P. acnes* and *S. epidermidis*.[111] While *P. acnes* is usually involved in the maintenance of healthy skin, especially within the oily skin follicles, it can also act as an opportunistic pathogen.[108] When skin microflora is stable or in a state of symbiosis, *S. epidermidis* interacts with and inhibits the overgrowth of *P. acnes*. However, a shift triggered by health, lifestyle or environmental changes can increase the activity and colonization of *P. acnes* within the follicles of the skin. This buildup reduces microbial diversity and creates a pathogenic coating or "biofilm" that further contributes to the severity of the acne.[109] Typical treatment approaches include topical and oral antibiotics to calm inflammation and pathogen overgrowth. However, antibiotics have been proven to wipe out good and bad microbes alike. Plus, *P. acnes* can also become resistant to antibiotics!

Side effects from chronic antibiotic use and other treatment options have caused experts to seek out alternative and natural approaches for acne-prone skin.[110] With an increased focus on the skin microbiome, the use of bacteria to combat and manage acne is promising. Taken orally, probiotics are proving beneficial either alone or along with typically prescribed medications.[111] In human clinical trials, probiotic supplements helped to clear the skin and visibly reduce the appearance of acne. Researchers propose that probiotics may help limit inflammation and oxidative

stress, control sebum production, rebalance gut microflora, and restore skin barrier function and hydration when used as a dietary supplement.[112] In one study, half of the patients took an oral supplement containing 250 milligrams of *L. acidophilus* and *B. bifidum* in conjunction with standard care and reported better outcomes compared to the non-probiotic supplemented group.[113] Another trial compared the use of probiotics either combined with or without the antibiotic minocycline. The researchers concluded that probiotics should be considered as an option for acne management because of their anti-inflammatory effect and ability to reduce potential adverse effects that come from chronic antibiotic use.[114] A different study revealed that a fermented dairy beverage containing Lactobacillus led to significant decreases in total acne lesions and helped to control sebum production when consumed over 12 weeks.[115] In 2018, researchers evaluated the effects of a prebiotic supplement on a small group of females with adult acne. After three months of supplementing with prebiotics (with no other changes in diet and lifestyle), improvements in glycemic control indirectly helped improve the subjects' skin conditions.[116]

Thanks to these studies, we know that erratic blood sugar and insulin levels, inflammation and oxidative stress have been linked to the development of acne. We also know that supplemented probiotics and prebiotics (known as synbiotics) reduce systemic oxidative stress and inflammation, indirectly improving the appearance of adult acne. These types of studies continue to show that the skin does not work in isolation. What we consume affects our skin, and even has the potential to restore and balance our skin's health.

Certain topical probiotics and bacterial strains can also be helpful in restoring health for acne-prone skin. Human and in-vitro studies show that when applied topically, probiotics help equalize skin microflora and barrier function, control inflammation, and

provide antimicrobial effects on blemishes.[117] For example, when *S. epidermidis*, which acne-prone skin lacks, was applied topically to blemishes, it inhibited and repelled *P. acnes* through a process of fermentation.[118] This study was the first to show how bacterial interference can control microbe predominance and improve skin conditions.

Different probiotic lactic acid bacteria can also provide benefits to manage acne.[119] One trial showed more than a 50 percent reduction in acne inflammation after eight weeks of topical application of the probiotic *Enterococcus faecalis*.[120] A different seven-day trial found that when applied topically, the probiotic strain *Streptococcus thermophiles* increased the subjects' production of ceramides[121] (lipids that help form the skin barrier and help retain it's moisture). The increased ceramide production strengthened the subjects' skin barriers, restored their skin's healthy, stabilizing fats, and had antimicrobial effects on blemishes. In another study, the probiotic strain *S. salivarius* was found to inhibit skin inflammation common to acne.[122]

The effect of prebiotics on acne-prone skin is also being investigated in clinical trials. One study used sucrose as a prebiotic fuel source for resident bacterium *S. epidermidis*, which was then applied to blemishes. Applying sucrose on blemished areas restored microbial balance, controlled the overgrowth of *P. acnes* and cleared the skin.[123]

ATOPIC DERMATITIS AND ECZEMA (MOIST SKIN)

Atopic dermatitis is a condition that creates uncomfortable and scratchy skin that may be red or flaky in appearance. It is important to note that atopic dermatitis and eczema are slightly

different, but they are often used interchangeably, or as general terms to describe many types of skin inflammation.

As we have learned, microbes communicate with our immune system to regulate and protect us against harmful pathogens from our environment. Microbial diversity is also important for maintaining a balanced and healthy skin microbiome. In atopic dermatitis, there is less diversity of generally healthy bacteria on the skin.[124] This dysbiosis is thought to be the driving force behind atopic dermatitis and calls for new approaches in treatment options.[125] A systematic review of 17 published studies found that atopic dermatitis was associated with very low microbial diversity and an overabundance of *Staphylococcus aureus* and *Staphylococcus epidermidis*. The researchers confirmed that the state of dysbiosis within skin microflora was a major factor contributing to atopic dermatitis.[126] In addition, epidemiological studies have shown food allergies, our modern approaches to skincare and excess cleansing (the "hygiene hypothesis") are also contributing factors to the progression of atopic dermatitis.[127]

Using knowledge of the skin microbiome and addressing the effects of microbial dysbiosis on conditions such as atopic dermatitis opens up promising new directions for management and treatment options. In 2015, a panel of Canadian dermatologists exploring the role of the skin microbiome on atopic dermatitis agreed that:

1. In atopic patients, the skin microbiome of affected skin lesions is different from unaffected skin areas;

2. Worsening atopic dermatitis and lower bacterial diversity are strongly associated; and

3. Application of products containing a combination of antioxidant and antibacterial components may increase microbiome diversity in atopic skin.[128]

Restoring gut and skin microflora with probiotics has been studied in numerous human clinical trials with mixed results.[129] As trials evolve, evidence for the use of pre- and probiotics to alleviate symptoms of atopic dermatitis grows more and more promising. What remains in question is identifying the right mixture of species/strains, dosage and duration of use for the most effective care.[130] One particular study looked at the synbiotic mixture of seven strains of probiotic bacteria and prebiotic fructo-oligosaccharide (FOS) in infants and children aged three months to six years with atopic dermatitis. They concluded that the blend of probiotics and FOS clinically improved the severity of the children's condition.[131] Dietary or probiotic supplements regulate inflammatory and/or hyperallergic responses, which benefits gut microflora and subsequently soothes atopic skin conditions.[132]

PSORIASIS (DRY SKIN)

Psoriasis is most active on dry skin areas such as the elbows, knees and torso, where skin becomes red and scaly and has a plaque-like appearance. Psoriasis is an immune-mediated and inflammatory condition affecting 2 to 4 percent of the global population. In addition to its genetic predisposition, several environmental factors like bacterial infection and dysbiosis, antibiotic treatment, and diet can magnify the condition.[133] The role of bacteria, in particular streptococci (the bacterium that causes throat infections), was reported to be a potential trigger for psoriasis over half a century ago. In more recent years, it was found that psoriasis skin sites have less microbial diversity and a dysbiosis of health-promoting residential bacteria when compared to healthy skin.[134]

It has also been suggested that psoriasis plaques form due to an intolerance to certain microbes that cause rapid accumulation of skin cells.[135] Additional studies have suggested that several microorganisms are associated with psoriasis' exacerbation, including *Staphylococcus aureus* and Malassezia fungi.[136]

Rebalancing gut-skin microflora could be a promising option in managing psoriasis, especially with the probiotic *Lactobacillus*. Researchers found psoriatic patients who took a daily dosage of *Lactobacillus paracasei* had less skin sensitivity and improved skin barrier function and hydration. Alternatively, an animal study showed that *Lactobacillus pentosus* had the ability to depress inflammatory reactions associated with the skin condition.[137] Even altering one's diet has been found to help the appearance of psoriasis. Patients with the condition often have a gluten sensitivity or intolerance, and when a gluten-free diet was followed, their skin health and appearance improved.[138]

SENSITIVE OR REACTIVE SKIN

When you have sensitive or reactive skin, it can feel tight, burn, tingle or become red in appearance in response to almost anything. Impaired skin barrier, changes in skin pH, and dysbiosis within gut microflora can affect both skin's immune response and its microflora communities. These factors instigate sensitive skin reactions. The use of prebiotics applied topically could potentially ease sensitive skin because they have the ability to stimulate or reduce bacterial growth to reestablish microbial symbiosis. [139]When 40 healthy adult women consumed the prebiotic galacto-oligosaccharides alone or paired with probiotic *Bifidobacterium breve*, skin barrier and hydration were significantly improved within four weeks. It was also found that the synbiotic supplement

containing both pre- and probiotics alone decreased toxins within the gut that may cause disturbances to the skin.[140]

DANDRUFF

Dandruff affects about 50 percent of the global population and is influenced by three factors: sebum, microbial metabolism and dysbiosis. Your scalp is covered with sebaceous units that produce sebum and sweat glands that increase moisture. Sebum secretion rates tend to be highest in the teen years through the mid-30s and decline from there. Sebum is also a food source for the growth and activity of bacteria and fungi, which means that a surplus could affect the skin microflora on the scalp.[141] Dandruff occurs when there is overgrowth and activity of a group of fungi called Malassezia on the scalp. This fungi produces high levels of irritating fatty acids that stimulate skin cell production, causing scaling and flakiness.[142] When in dysbiosis, bacterial microbes can also aggravate dandruff.[143]

One clinical trial of 140 women looked at the bacterial and fungal diversity of the scalp microbiome and found the ratio of *Propionibacterium acnes* to *Staphylococcus epidermis* was higher on a healthy scalp compared to a scalp with dandruff. Moreover, bacteria may also be involved in supplying essential vitamins and amino acids for healthy hair and scalp, particularly biotin, vitamin B6, nicotinate and lysine. Conclusions from this and other studies suggest that products working to rebalance scalp microflora (particularly to enhance Propionibacterium activity while suppressing Staphylococcus activity) better manage and support a healthy scalp.[144]

With the importance of bacteria on the scalp microbiome, probiotics should be considered for future treatment options for dandruff. In a European study, the probiotic *Lactobacillus paracasei*

NCC 2461 (ST11) was supplemented on healthy men with moderate to severe dandruff. A significant improvement in scalp health with less inflammation was reported after 56 days of use. With no adverse effects, the study concluded that the probiotic's positive effect on dandruff is most likely due to reestablishing the skin barrier and skin immune system, which restored and balanced the scalp microbiome.[145]

From these studies, we know that dandruff develops from an imbalanced scalp microbiome, sebum overproduction and other factors, including changes in skin pH, hair product buildup and excessive washing. New and integrative approaches with a focus on probiotic supplements and topical shampoos could offer more promising results in restoring scalp health and minimizing the side effects of dandruff.

PHOTO AGING

We all know that the sun is bad for our skin. Additionally, as we age, our naturally occurring skin antioxidant defense system slows down and can become more easily overwhelmed by environmental stressors (as discussed in Chapter 3). Over time, visible effects of photo aging can include the development of fine lines and wrinkles, loss of skin tone and elasticity, decline in skin thickness and circulation, hyperpigmentation, inflamed and broken capillaries, and a loss in skin moisture.[146]

The effect of UV radiation (UVR) on the skin microbiome is less studied, but emerging evidence shows that different microorganisms may have particular sensitivities to UV rays. Our skin's microbes regularly communicate with immune receptors to maintain healthy skin. So when sun exposure weakens our skin's immune system, changes in skin microflora associated with UVR are also likely to occur. We now know that any shift in microbial

communities can disrupt equilibrium and negatively impact immune responses in the skin.[147]

The good news is that the use of probiotics looks promising as a potential option to slow skin aging and support skin immunity against chronic sun exposure.[148] In a human clinical trial, the probiotic *Lactobacillus johnsonii* along with a carotenoid antioxidant was taken by healthy women for 10 weeks. Compared to the non-supplemented group, the women taking the supplement showed faster skin recovery after sun exposure.[149] Another 12-week study on probiotic *Lactobacillus plantarum* HY7714 revealed significant improvements in skin hydration and elasticity with a reduction in wrinkle severity in women with dry, photo-aged skin.[150] Other probiotic strains including *Lactobacillus acidophilus* and *Lactobacillus rhamnosus* have also been proven effective in reducing or combating the aging effects caused by long-term sun exposure.[151]

As we learn the importance of microbes in the regulation of the skin's immune system, it only makes sense to further our understanding of the potential use of probiotics in combating skin stress associated with chronic sun exposure.

ROSACEA

Rosacea is associated with persistent flushing or redness of the skin. It is usually most prominent on the cheeks, nose or chin. Multiple factors may trigger rosacea, including an overload of Demodex mites and Malassezia fungi, which offset the skin ecosystem, and *Helicobacter pylori* infection within gut microflora. Irregular skin's fatty acid composition is also characteristic in rosacea. It leaves skin dry but also changes its microbial balance.[152]

Restoring balance within the gut and skin microbiome are important for rosacea. Including probiotic cultures such as Lactobacilli

and/or Bifidobacterium along with prebiotics and dietary changes could support conventional treatments and restore gut and skin health.[153]

Research on the skin microbiome is now just beginning to reveal the intricate relationship microbes have with the skin, gut and immune system in maintaining healthy skin. When microbes are in a state of dysbiosis, they can have a profound effect on skin immunity and metabolism, abetting the onset of certain skin conditions.

Either through dietary, supplement or topical intervention, pre- and probiotics may offer new and promising approaches that stabilize and nurture the skin to bring it back to a state of balance and optimal health.

Let's learn more about them in Chapter 5.

What You Should Know about Pre- and Probiotics

~~~

In the previous chapters we learned that we coexist with microbes that communicate continuously with our skin cells and immune system, supporting the health and preservation of our skin. We also learned that although there are a few main resident bacterial groups dominant on the skin, our own biochemical individuality and lifestyle diversifies the type and number of microbes that constitute our individual biome cloud.

In Chapter 4 we learned that pre- and probiotics can help support skin immunity and encourage the colonization of beneficial bacteria. Based on systematic reviews, oral therapy with pre- and probiotics (and even postbiotics, which we will learn about in this chapter) may prevent and treat atopic skin conditions in children and adults.[154]

Even though pre- and probiotics have become popular topics in recent years, there is still a lot of confusion about what they are and what to look for when reading the ingredients labels on food, drinks, dietary supplements and skincare products. In this chapter we will get down to some basics on pre- and probiotics so you can make informed choices.

COMMON PROBIOTICS

The term "probiotic" is derived from Greek, meaning "for life." It was then formally defined in the 1960s as "substances secreted by one microorganism that stimulate the growth of another." A decade later, the following was added to the definition: "organisms and substances that contribute to intestinal microbial balance." The modern definition of probiotics as agreed upon by the Food and Agriculture Organization of the United Nations and the World Health Organization states, "Live microorganisms which when administered in adequate amounts confer a health benefit to the host."[155]

We now know they naturally exist in and on the body, but they can also be consumed through diet and supplementation or applied to the skin.

Some common probiotic microorganisms that may be used in foods, beverages, supplements, skincare and pharmaceuticals include:

Lactobacillus sp.	Bifidobacterium sp.	Enterococcus sp.	Streptococcus sp.
L. acidophilus	B. bifidum	E. faecalis	S. cremoris
L. casei	B. adolescentis	E. faecium	S. salivarius
L. delbrueckii ssp. (bulgaricus)	B. animalis		S. diacetylactis
L. cellobiosus	B. infantis		S. intermedius
L. curvatus	B. thermophilum		
L. fermentum	B. longum		
L. lactis			
L. plantarum			
L. reuteri			
L. rhamnosus			
L. brevis			
L. johnsonii			
L. gasseri			
L. pentosus			

GENERAL HEALTH BENEFITS OF PROBIOTICS

Probiotics offer a wide variety of health benefits, including;

❋ Normalizing intestinal health by balancing pH, promoting healthy gut microflora, detoxifying/neutralizing harmful pathogens, and improving the absorption and bioavailability of nutrients from diet and supplements.

❋ Strengthening and balancing the immune system to regulate inflammation and allergic responses in the body.

❋ Produce and increase bioavailability of nutrients.

❋ Support weight management and metabolism health.

Good Bacteria for Healthy Skin

* Via the gut-brain axis, support mental health including emotional stress or depressed mood.

* Balance and support skin health.[156]

PROBIOTICS FOR HEALTHY SKIN

Probiotic microorganisms can improve the well-being of our skin when consumed orally or applied as a topical. A growing body of clinical evidence shows that these microbes have the ability to enhance the health and appearance of our skin.[157] You can see in Figure 5.1 the various ways probiotics can help your skin microbiome.

FIGURE 5.1: HOW PROBIOTICS HELP CREATE HEALTHY SKIN

BY DIETARY MEANS	BY TOPICAL APPLICATION
• Modifies and regulates skin immunity, inflammation • Helps reduce hyperactive immune responses associated with allergens or chronic skin conditions • Has antioxidant properties, protecting skin from environmental aggressors and pollutants • Neutralizes harmful pathogens in the gut, before they reach skin tissue	• Has antibacterial and antimicrobial effects • Promotes healthy skin barrier function and natural moisturizing • Supports skin cell renewal • Stimulates skin's natural antimicrobial defense • Controls inflammation • Assists in wound healing or infection

Through dietary and/or topical means, probiotics support skin health by:

* Protecting against environmental aggressors and pollutants.

* Balancing skin microflora to promote a state of symbiosis.

* Detoxifying and preventing the overgrowth of harmful pathogens from dietary or topical exposure.

* Providing anti-inflammatory and anti-allergic effects for sensitive and chronic skin conditions.

* Strengthening the skin barrier, stimulating ceramide production and locking in skin moisture.

* Producing and/or providing nutrients for the "good" skin microbes to flourish and maintain healthy skin.[158]

Now that we know some of the amazing benefits probiotics can offer, let's learn a little bit more about how they are regulated and how to decipher them on a label.

PROBIOTICS REGULATORY CONFUSION: NOVEL FOOD? DIETARY SUPPLEMENT? PHARMACEUTICAL?

A number of probiotic products are available on the international market as food supplements, dietary supplements, natural health products, functional foods and medicinal foods/supplements. The position and regulation of probiotics has become confusing because they are moderated independently in different countries. Therefore, when choosing a probiotic product, it is important to be aware of the sourcing, manufacturing and packaging of the product from an overall safety and efficacy perspective, in addition to the specific health benefit or claim.[159]

Canada is one of the most progressive countries in regulating and approving specific health claims of probiotics to date.

Furthermore, to help health experts and consumers make informed choices on probiotic products, Canada developed a clinical guide and approval list for those commercially available probiotics that met the following inclusion criteria:

* Generally Recognized as Safe status in the U.S. (FDA) and/or Natural Product Number (Health Canada) for probiotic strain(s) used in the products.

* Favorable published clinical evidence for the particular strain(s) present in each product.

* For products containing multiple strains, evidence must be for the specified combination and *not* extrapolated from the evidence for the separate probiotic strains.[160]

PROBIOTICS—HOW THEY WORK AND WHAT TO LOOK FOR ON A LABEL

Because there are so many different types of probiotics available on the market, what follows is a general example of what a product or supplement label could look like. Some labels may provide proprietary blends (as referenced here), but some countries may require that each strain state the exact amount of colony-forming units (CFUs) on the label. Obviously, the more you know about the probiotic, the better. So I always recommend that you research the ingredients, manufacturer and health claims, as well as the research behind those claims. If you compare different companies and their products, what you may find is the most transparent labels often have gone through rigorous processes to produce a credible and high-quality product for the market. Most times, it's worth a little investigation!

Here's an example of how to read a probiotic supplement label:

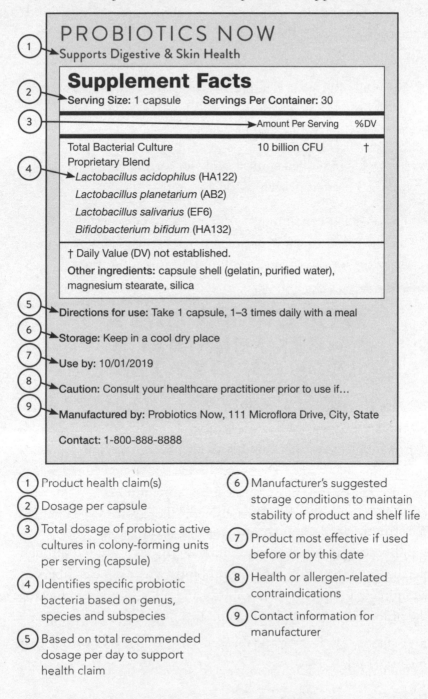

① Product health claim(s)

② Dosage per capsule

③ Total dosage of probiotic active cultures in colony-forming units per serving (capsule)

④ Identifies specific probiotic bacteria based on genus, species and subspecies

⑤ Based on total recommended dosage per day to support health claim

⑥ Manufacturer's suggested storage conditions to maintain stability of product and shelf life

⑦ Product most effective if used before or by this date

⑧ Health or allergen-related contraindications

⑨ Contact information for manufacturer

HOW ARE PROBIOTICS MADE
FOR COMMERCIAL USE?

The commercial production of probiotics is challenging, technical and requires many steps to ensure the probiotic strain is isolated, living and stable for distribution and sale. These bacteria are derived from varied food and natural sources, then grown and processed for safe consumption under regulated manufacturing conditions. Probiotics are very susceptible to environmental factors such as oxygen, processing and preservation methods, acidity, and salt concentration, which collectively affect their overall viability.[161]

When put into product form, they can be suspended in liquids or powders that involve different steps in processing. Let's take powdered forms, for example. The following steps would be processed under tightly regulated and quality-controlled conditions:

1. Grow and ferment the bacteria from dairy or nondairy mediums.

2. Centrifuge the blend to separate and isolate the bacteria from the food blend.

3. Freeze-dry the probiotic strain to remove excess moisture or oxygen.

From there, additional steps can be taken to protect the bacteria cell structure and viability, such as coating the capsule to improve stability of the product even when ingested and processed through the digestive tract.[162] Storing the probiotic with prebiotic fibers or vitamin C can help improve stability and offers a source of fuel for the probiotic to remain active and "alive."

Probiotics have a shorter shelf life compared to most dietary supplements, but can remain active and stabilize their cell count by

about 90 percent for one year. Moreover, new manufacturing techniques are improving their shelf life, with some proposing stability for up to two years. Once the package is opened, probiotics should be used within one to three months.

THE REAL CHALLENGE FOR PROBIOTICS—SURVIVING THE STRESS TEST (YOUR DIGESTION)

In order to be effective, probiotic strains must withstand the digestive enzymes, low pH, gastric juices and bile salts during the digestive process. A probiotic must have the ability to survive in the gut and adhere to the intestinal tract in order to exert its health benefits. Digestive resistance varies among different probiotic strains. For example, Lactobacillus is more resilient in a low-pH environment than Bifidobacteria genus. Live probiotic strains that can withstand or resist the abrasive digestive environment and stick to and colonize along the digestive tract will have the ability to exert their health-promoting effects.[163]

As they travel through the intestinal tract, probiotics flourish and interact with resident microbes. Their influence on our gut microbiota and immune system ultimately affects the health of our skin.

HOW ARE THEY CLASSIFIED?

A probiotic bacterium is recognized by the group (genus), species, subspecies (if applicable), and an alphanumeric designation identifying a specific strain.[164]

Using a strain designation system not only helps to identify the probiotic, but also provides insight on their unique properties, mechanisms and health-promoting effects.[165]

DOSAGE AND LABELING—
COLONY-FORMING WHAT?

One of the major inconsistencies among probiotics is how they're labeled on a product. You may notice some probiotic labels reference metric unit milligrams (mg), which is based on weight. Others refer to the number of colony-forming units (CFU), which is the amount or number of viable, live active bacteria in the product upon production. Most countries require ingredients to be labeled by weight, which has created industry inconsistencies and consumer confusion. It's important to know that, when reading the label of a probiotic product, *it is the number of active microorganisms providing the health benefit, not the milligrams or weight of the probiotic provided*. Because of this, in 2018 the Food and Drug Administration released a draft guidance document approving CFUs as a unit of measure for probiotics on labels. When seeking out a good-quality probiotic, make sure you're looking at total CFUs and the combination of probiotic strains versus the milligram amount.[166] As recommended by a leading academic association, the International Scientific Association of Probiotics and Prebiotics (ISAPP), most effective probiotic doses range from 100 million to 50 billion or more CFUs per dose.[167]

NOT ALL PROBIOTICS ARE CREATED EQUAL

A range of factors can affect a probiotic's effectiveness, from manufacturing temperatures to surviving digestion and adhering to the intestinal tract or sticking to the skin when applied topically. Different strains vary in their effectiveness as well. If you're seeking a probiotic to support skin health for example, look for foods, supplements or skincare products that offer those specific strains with skin health claims (see page 82). Also look at symbiotic blends that may include a variety of strains along with prebiotics to strengthen product effectiveness.

ARE PROBIOTICS SAFE?

According to leading health associations and evidence from clinical trials, probiotics are generally safe to consume. If supplementing, be sure to read the label and follow the directions for use. For example, if you are pregnant, have an autoimmune condition or short bowel syndrome, ISAPP suggests consulting your healthcare practitioner before using a probiotic product.[168]

HOW SHOULD PROBIOTICS BE STORED?

Check the label for recommended storage requirements. Depending on the type and manufacturing process, some probiotics don't need refrigeration. If refrigeration is not required, store them in a cool dry place. Remember, probiotics are living microbes, so you want to protect them and maximize their shelf life.

WHAT ABOUT POSTBIOTICS?

Although manufacturing technologies are improving, some of the challenges around the bioavailability, stability and shelf life of probiotics have caused experts to take notice of postbiotics. Postbiotics are non-living byproducts from by probiotic microorganisms that have benefit the host.[169] They may include bacteriocins, organic acids, ethanol, diacetyl, acetaldehydes and hydrogen peroxide, and offer anti-pathogenic properties or have even been suggested to stimulate skin collagen production and support a healthy skin barrier.[170] As a probiotic breaks down or dies off in a supplement or skincare product, these metabolites become present as well within the product. Research on postbiotics suggests that these non-viable byproducts could potentially become active ingredients in future formulations because of their enhanced stability and potential health benefits. Be on the lookout for postbiotics as this market evolves!

PREBIOTICS

Though probiotics and prebiotics sound alike, they are actually different, which means how they function in and on the body is different as well. Prebiotics are not bacteria. Rather, they are undigestible dietary fibers that feed the good bacteria that live inside the large intestine or on the skin.[171] The most commonly studied prebiotics are fructans (fructo-oligosaccharides, or FOS, and inulin) and galactans (galacto-oligosaccharides, or GOS). Both have the ability to enrich probiotics Lactobacillus and Bifidobacterium within the digestive tract. Other well-known prebiotics include oligofructose and lactulose.[172]

Prebiotics are carbohydrate fibers that have a positive effect on and can modify the gut and skin microbiota. Through the fermentation of prebiotics by gut and skin microorganisms, prebiotics provide a major source of energy for good bacteria and play a significant role in enriching the activity and colonization of health-promoting bacteria within the gut and on the skin.[173]

NATURAL SOURCES OF PREBIOTICS

Prebiotic	Dietary Sources
Fructo-oligosaccharides (FOS)	Onions, leeks, asparagus, chicory, Jerusalem artichoke, garlic, oats
Inulin	Agave, banana, chicory, dandelion, garlic, globe and Jerusalem artichokes, onion, wild yam
Isomalto-oligosaccharides	Miso, soy sauce, sake, honey
Lactulose	Skim milk
Lactosucrose	Milk sugar
Galacto-oligosaccharides	Lentil, chickpeas, green peas, lima beans, kidney beans

Soybean oligosaccharides	Soybeans
Xylo-oligosaccharides	Bamboo shoots, fruits, vegetables, milk, honey
Arabinoxylan oligosaccharides	Bran of grasses (cereal grains)
Resistant Starch	Beans/legumes, starchy fruits and vegetables (plantains, bananas, sweet potatoes, corn), whole grains

Prebiotics help those good bacteria (probiotics) flourish and maintain a state of symbiosis within the gut and skin microbiota. They also help microbes produce health-promoting metabolites such as short-chain fatty acids that can boost the immune system and improve the bioavailability of dietary minerals including iron, calcium and magnesium. Moreover, prebiotics have been found to support bone health, help to manage inflammation and promote a healthy metabolism.[174] Based on these combined health effects, the ISAPP defines prebiotics as "a substrate that is selectively utilized by host microorganisms conferring a health benefit"[175] You can think of them as a source of fuel for microbes. When bacteria are sufficiently fueled with prebiotics, they in turn are able to flourish, protect and maintain a state of balance or as we know now "symbiosis."

Although all prebiotics can be classified as fibers, not all fibers are prebiotic. In order for a fiber to qualify as a "prebiotic" it must have the following properties:

※ Insoluble or partially soluble within the digestive tract

※ Resists digestive acidity, enzymes and absorption in the upper GI tract

※ Well fermented by beneficial intestinal bacteria

✱ Stimulates the growth and/or activity of intestinal bacteria associated with promoting health and well-being.[176]

Since there are many forms and sources of prebiotics found in foods, it shouldn't be challenging to get enough of them, but how much is enough? Experts propose we should consume them more often to attain their health benefits (about 5 grams of prebiotic fiber per day, rather than the 2 to 3 grams generally consumed in the modern diet).[177] Prebiotics can be easily consumed from food, functional foods (a food that has specific nutrients added to it to offer a potentially positive health effect beyond the basic diet), powders and dietary supplements, but remember they're a form of fiber, so increase your intake slowly and ensure you hydrate as well to minimize digestive upset. Most plant-based foods are great sources of fiber, and some are more concentrated with prebiotics.

You can boost your dietary prebiotic intake by eating high-fiber cereals, whole grains, fruits, vegetables, nuts, seeds and legumes. Some top choices include:

✱ *Vegetables*—Jerusalem artichoke, chicory, garlic, leeks, onions, shallots, cabbage

✱ *Legumes*—chickpeas, lentils, red kidney beans, baked beans, soybeans

✱ *Fruits*—bananas, watermelon, grapefruit

✱ *Cereal grains*—bran, barley, oats

✱ *Nuts and seeds*—almonds, pistachios, flaxseeds

Also, if you're on a specialized diet such as a low-FODMAP diet (a type of diet low in fermentable carbohydrates that may be clinically recommended for the management of irritable bowel syndrome), consult your healthcare practitioner before considering a prebiotic-

rich diet.[178] We will discuss more on getting prebiotics through diet in the next chapter as well.

HOW PREBIOTICS WORK FOR HEALTHY SKIN

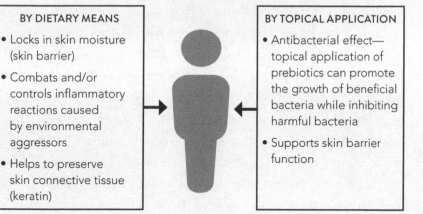

BY DIETARY MEANS

- Locks in skin moisture (skin barrier)
- Combats and/or controls inflammatory reactions caused by environmental aggressors
- Helps to preserve skin connective tissue (keratin)

BY TOPICAL APPLICATION

- Antibacterial effect— topical application of prebiotics can promote the growth of beneficial bacteria while inhibiting harmful bacteria
- Supports skin barrier function

PREBIOTICS FOR HEALTHY SKIN

Prebiotics have emerged in recent years as potentially effective dietary and topical ingredients to support skin health. Initial clinical studies observed that prebiotics helped calm allergic or immune-related skin conditions, such as atopic dermatitis. More recent studies have found that certain prebiotics either alone or in combination with probiotics can help lessen skin stress and inflammatory reactions associated with sun exposure. They can also improve skin's water retention and skin barrier function, and protect collagen and keratin, the key structural proteins in skin, from weakening and loss of tissue.[179]

SYNBIOTICS: THE SYNERGY EFFECT OF PRE- AND PROBIOTICS

Within the gut, probiotics are most active in the small and large intestine, while prebiotics are detected mainly in the large intestine. Together they work to promote healthy gut flora. When probiotics

and prebiotics are combined within functional foods (foods with concentrated health-promoting ingredients), supplements or even skincare products, these mixtures are called synbiotics. There are indications in clinical studies that with the addition of dietary prebiotics, dietary probiotics have a higher tolerance and stability within the intestinal tract. So, by combining them, there is an improved sustainability for probiotics to work effectively to balance and improve gut and skin microbiota.[180] Carefully selected prebiotics with probiotic strains must be considered to ensure that the prebiotic can effectively stimulate the growth and stability of the particular probiotic bacterium.

Some commonly used synbiotic mixtures include:

* Lactobacillus genus bacteria + inulin (often sourced from chicory root)

* Lactobacillus, Streptococcus and Bifidobacterium genus bacteria + fructo-oligosaccharides (FOS)

* Lactobacillus, Bifidobacterium, Enterococcus genus bacteria + FOS

* Lactobacillus and Bifidobacterium genus bacteria + oligofructose

* Lactobacillus and Bifidobacterium genus bacteria + inulin[181]

Clinical trials have shown synbiotics are useful in increasing Lactobacillus and Bifidobacterium bacteria within the gut and balancing the gut microbiota. Synbiotics have a variety of other beneficial properties, including antibacterial, detoxification, weight management, blood sugar balance, immune support and anti-allergenic effects.[182]

In one study of the treatment of atopic dermatitis in 40 infants and children, researchers combined seven probiotic strains with prebiotic FOS. After eight weeks of using the synbiotic supplement, clinically significant improvements were found in the severity of the skin condition for the children and infants treated.[183] This shows how synbiotics may offer superior results to rebalance and promote healthy skin, over pre- or probiotics used alone.

PROBIOTICS IN SKINCARE

As people gain interest in the skin microbiome, probiotics are popping up everywhere in skin- and haircare products. These products promise that administering good bacteria to the skin's surface can combat blemishes, ward off wrinkles, eliminate dandruff and replenish moisture. As we learned in Chapter 3, overcleansing and the use of certain personal care products and fragrances can alter the skin microbiota. So including "good bacteria" in skincare makes sense, right?

Right. However, it is critical to understand how probiotics can help the skin when applied topically, because different strains will provide unique skin benefits (similar to when we ingest them by dietary or supplement means). In other words, if you're considering a probiotic in your skincare regimen, what exactly are you looking to get out of it?

Although the research on topical use of probiotics is not as advanced as dietary studies, certain probiotic extracts may provide anti-inflammatory, anti-microbial, pH balancing, anti-aging and moisturizing properties when applied to the surface of the skin.[184]

To work effectively on the skin, a probiotic must adhere or "stick" to the skin in order to provide any benefit. For example, an in vitro study found probiotic strains that adhered better to skin

keratin cells included *Lactobacillus acidophilus* LA-5, *Lactobacillus delbrueckii*, *Lactobacillus acidophilus*, LA-10, *Lactobacillus paracasei* LA-26, and *Bifidobacterium lactis* B-94 and Bb12.[185] Once a probiotic can stick to the skin, it has the ability to control pathogenic overgrowth and/or replenish skin microbiota and health. Probiotics can also create metabolites, postbiotics or bio-actives (compounds that may offer a skin health benefit beyond probiotics) that benefit the skin, including:

※ Organic acids (acetic and lactic acids) that help to lower and rebalance skin pH (to combat pathogen overgrowth), regulate inflammation and enhance skin's moisturization properties (*L. acidophilus* LA-10 and *L. paracasei* L-26).

※ Hyaluronic acid to support skin barrier function, moisture and tissue repair (*L. rhamnosus* FTDC 8313 and *L. gasseri* FTDC 8131).

※ Sphingomyelinase, an enzyme essential for ceramide production (*S. thermophilus*).

※ Lipoteichoic acid, a structural component of bacteria that has been found to stimulate skin defense and control inflammation when it comes from beneficial probiotics such as *L. plantarum* KCTC10887BP (*pLTA*).[186]

Sounds amazing, right? But wait, there's one more thing to think about. Because of the rapid growth of probiotics in the personal care market, some dermatologists and industry experts have challenged their overall efficacy in topical products. While countries are seeking to adopt more formal regulations and expand their understanding of topical probiotics through research, there are still serious questions to consider. Dr. Linda Katz, a dermatologist who presented at the 2018 Skin Microbiome Congress in Boston, asked some of these questions, such as:

✳ Are probiotics living or viable in topical products?

✳ What is their intended function or benefit in the product?

✳ Because they are a bacterium, how are they regulated and compared against microbial contamination testing?

✳ How can they be standardized and regulated across varying countries?[187]

Remember, probiotics are live microorganisms that are present within or on the body and that can be consumed or applied to the skin. They offer a wide range of positive health benefits through their influence on the immune system and maintaining microbial balance within the gut and skin. As a source of fuel for probiotics, prebiotic fibers help good bacteria flourish and counteract harmful microbes to maintain healthy gut and skin microbiota. When they're appropriately combined in functional foods, supplements or skincare products, they may provide stronger health benefits by working in synergy with one another.

Effects of Probiotics on Skin Health (Oral and/or Topical Use)[188]

Probiotics	Potential Skin Benefit Based on Clinical Evidence
Bifidobacteria species	Associated with immune regulation and reducing skin sensitivity
Lactobacillus acidophilus	Clinical improvement of acne
Lactobacillus bulgaricus	Clinical improvement of acne
Lactobacillus plantarum	Controls or calms skin inflammation
Lactobacillus delbreuckii	Remedy or treatment option for management of atopic dermatitis. Decreases skin sensitivity

Probiotics	Potential Skin Benefit Based on Clinical Evidence
Lactobacillus paracasei	Supports skin barrier function Remedy or treatment option for management of atopic dermatitis
Lactobacillus rhamnosus	Helps to protect against UV-induced/ environmental stressors Remedy or treatment option for management of atopic dermatitis
Lactobacillus reuteri	Protection of epidermal keratinocytes (predominant cell type in skin's outermost layer, the epidermis)
Lactobacillus salivarius	Remedy or treatment option for management of atopic dermatitis

When you're researching a probiotic-based product, here are five elements to consider:

1. Suggested Use—How do I use the product for best results? What are the product's claims? Are there any health-related contraindications I should be aware of?

2. Strain(s)—Look for appropriate strains related to the product's claims (i.e., anti-aging, dry or sensitive skin or certain skin conditions). Are the claims realistic? Are they clinically validated? For dietary products, look for the number of CFUs rather than milligrams (mg).

3. Science—Does the manufacturer provide clinical backing for the ingredients and formula? Is this a company-driven marketing study or is it backed by a study that is clinically validated, peer reviewed and published in a recognized medical or health-related journal? Is the product recognized by third-party qualified health experts or accredited associations?

4. Stability—What is the shelf life or expiration date on the product label? How should it be stored for ideal shelf life and product efficacy?

5. Seal Approval—Is the product produced within a regulated and qualified manufacturing facility, such as the goods and manufacturing practices (GMP)? Are there any third-party tests and certification seals on the packaging?

As we're learning, the skin does not work in isolation; rather, it is constantly interacting within your body, environment and the microbes we expose it to. Pre- and probiotics through diet, supplementation or topical application could help keep the skin clear, luminous and resilient against harmful pathogens or environmental aggressors that our skin is exposed to every day.

Now that you understand pre- and probiotics' contribution to and importance for healthy skin, we can now look at ways to utilize them and implement them more often into your daily lifestyle.

CHAPTER 6

Microbe-Friendly Nutrition

~~~

Your skin is a mirror image of your inner health and well-being. In the beginning of this book we learned about the gut-skin axis and how both components contain enormous microbial communities that communicate via immune, hormonal and neurotransmitter receptor pathways. Though they communicate indirectly, the microbiota within the gut and skin are a fully integrated system and their function and balance is essential for our overall health and well-being. Taking into account the gut-skin axis, it makes sense that what we put into our stomachs also affects our skin.

As a nutritionist, I often say that our health is largely influenced by the following three things:

1. The nutrients we consume.

2. How well those nutrients are digested and absorbed.

3. How well our bodies neutralize and eliminate pollutants.

If these three elements are routinely out of sync, then it is certain to show on your skin. And that's what's amazing about the healthy microorganisms and prebiotics we have been discussing in this book! By nurturing your microbiome from the inside and out, with sound nutrition and lifestyle choices, these flourishing and healthy gut microbial communities will promote a healthy body that will influence the appearance and health of your skin.

HOW GOOD NUTRITION PROMOTES HEALTHY SKIN

The link between nutrition and the skin is showing up more and more, from grocery store aisles to skincare and makeup brands promoting "beauty from within." The notion of "hope in a jar" has shifted away from covering up flaws or reversing aging and toward preventative and more holistic ways to nurture and care for our skin. Now hardly a day passes that there isn't a headline about something intriguing (or oversensationalized) on the topic.

Do you remember in Chapter 2 when we discussed the basic physiology of the skin? New skin cells are produced in those deeper, dermal layers of skin and pushed up toward the outer epidermal layer. If we are well-nourished and our digestion is working properly, nutrients can reach those dermal layers via the bloodstream. There they encourage healthy skin cell renewal and defend and support the skin's structural integrity. Generally new skin cells are formed every three to four weeks, but the natural process of aging, poor diet and a toxic lifestyle slow down skin cell metabolism. When skin cell metabolism is slow, new, revitalized skin cells take longer to reach the outer epidermal layer. This leads

to a dull, uneven complexion and a buildup of dead surface skin. It's important to exfoliate our skin to remove debris and surface buildup, but it's just as important to consider what you're putting into your body for the health of your skin. For best health, your skin needs nourishment and care from the inside and outside.

YOU ARE WHAT YOU CONSUME, METABOLIZE AND FLOURISH

When you think about what we have learned about the skin micro-biome—what it is, how it works and adapts with our bodies from the inside and from the outside—it's amazing to think of the huge impact that teeny tiny microbes have on our overall health and well-being. Interestingly, the microbiome is a driving force behind the industry of personalized nutrition. There are at-home testing methods that you can do yourself to assess your gut microbiota. Based on the results, you can tailor a nutritional and supplemental program to fit your current health status and future goals. Pretty cool stuff!

While "you are what you eat," you may also hear the saying "you are what you eat and metabolize," meaning that although you could be following a nutritionally balanced diet, if your digestive system is not functioning well, then nutrients are not efficiently processed and bioavailable to the body. Makes sense, right? Now let me propose that "you are what you eat, metabolize *and flourish*." Now that you have learned about caring for the good bacteria that lives inside you and on your skin, I hope this makes as much sense to you as it does to me.

BEAUTIFY YOUR SKIN BIOME WITH MICROBE-FRIENDLY NUTRITION

Nutrition is probably one of the most convoluted yet overgeneralized topics out there today. I'm sure you've been in conversations or overheard questions like: Which diet is best? What foods should or shouldn't I be eating? How often or when do I eat or avoid them? Which cleanse should I try? With the plethora of information available it can be confusing to know what is credible over what is purely a marketing ploy. But this is also the beauty of nutrition (no pun intended) and why I love it! It is constantly evolving and sparking intriguing conversation and debate. I have an integrated background in nutritional sciences, natural health and personal care and still learn something new every day. I know how confusing nutrition can be. That's why I've created a plan that encourages you to make changes that are realistic and achievable.

We're all unique—your age, bio-individuality, lifestyle and environment need to be considered so you can successfully achieve your personal skin health goals. When working with my clients, I often use the 80/20 rule because I've seen them get the most positive, attainable and long-term results that way. Without complete restriction, a change in habit followed most of the time (80 percent) will incur more positive and long-lasting results. Obviously the more you practice a new habit, the better the result, but remember that it's okay to be gentle with yourself! This plan is about supporting your individual needs while making modifications in your diet and lifestyle to promote a state of symbiosis. Some of these modifications may be more difficult to follow than others, so take your time and allow wiggle room to discover what works best for you.

So, with all you now know about how pre- and probiotics can affect your skin health, what can you eat to help these microbes

remain balanced and happy? And what is microbe-friendly nutrition exactly? With the importance of microbial symbiosis for the health and sensitivity of our skin *and* its bio-communitive relationship with the gut, this plan works to purify, nurture and balance skin health through foods that detoxify harmful microbes while encouraging good skin bacteria to flourish for a balanced gut and skin microbiota.

MICROBE-FRIENDLY NUTRITION— DIETARY CONSIDERATIONS

There is an incredible relationship that exists between food and our microbiome. Early studies discovered that different cultural diets influence gut microbes, and there is continued interest in understanding how certain dietary components affect the gut microbiota, the body and the skin. For instance, we now know how modern and Western diets negatively impact microbes' normal function in the gut. On the flip side, certain foods and diets have proven to have the ability to nurture and balance gut microbiota.

Diets relying heavily on vegetables and fruits contribute to a healthy and balanced digestive system. Packed with antioxidants and anti-inflammatory properties, vegetables and fruits also influence the microbes in your gut.[189] A good example of this is the Mediterranean diet, which promotes longevity and supports skin health.[190] It has been one of my go-to foundational diets when developing beauty-infused skin nutrition programs and products over the years.

Why do I like it? The traditional Mediterranean diet is high in vegetables, fruits, nuts, legumes and unrefined cereals; healthy fats from virgin olive oil in salads, cooked vegetables and legumes; moderate amounts of fish and shellfish; a low consumption

of meat and meat products; and even allows for a glass of wine during meals! Fermented dairy products (cheese and yogurt) can also be consumed in sensible amounts. Rich in antioxidants and bioactive components with anti-inflammatory effects, it has a low glycemic index and is a good source of prebiotics because of its high fiber content.[191] The diet also provides a variety of pre- and probiotic-rich foods, which makes it a great starting point for microbe-friendly nutrition.

However, with our modern, fast-paced lifestyle, it is easy to oversimplify the true traditional practices of the Mediterranean diet. Here are some ways to more easily and correctly adapt to the diet's traditional principles.

PRACTICAL WAYS TO INCORPORATE MEDITERRANEAN DIETARY PRINCIPLES

* Olive oil—Use extra-virgin or virgin olive oil on vegetables and legumes in salads, stir fries and sautés. Pair with herbs, spices, garlic, onion and lemon for flavor.

* Vegetables—Incorporate into lunch and dinner as part of main dish. At least one serving of vegetables every day should be raw. Top with olive oil, vinegar, lemon and herbs for salad dressings.

* Whole grains—Switch to high-fiber whole grain over white breads, pastas, rice and flour.

* Legumes—Consume three or more servings per week from a variety of beans, lentils, chickpeas and peas.

* Fish/seafood—Aim to get one or more servings per week of white fish (cod, flounder) and two or more servings of fatty fish (salmon, sardines, tuna) along with occasional shellfish

(oysters, clams, shrimp, squid). Wild-caught, fresh, frozen or canned are all options.

✳ Meat/poultry—Choose lean poultry over red meat. Moderate portion sizes (3 to 4 ounces) and frequency of consumption.[192]

Considering a change in your diet can be overwhelming at times, I would encourage you to look to the Mediterranean diet as a basis for microbe-friendly nutrition. Use it as a quick guide and reference to keep you on track. We will come back to it at the end of this chapter. Now, I want to continue to discuss ways to purify, nurture and balance the gut-skin microbiome with nutrition. First we will focus on macronutrients that support the health of our skin.

THE MACRONUTRIENTS

We obtain a large portion of our energy and nutrients from the three macronutrients: proteins, fats and carbohydrates. We know that the balance and proportion of the three is important for optimal health, but it has also been found that the types of protein, fat and carbohydrates can influence the balance and activity of gut microflora (and ultimately the skin).

PROTEINS

Studies have confirmed that the source of protein has a direct effect on your gut microbes and their overall diversity.[193] This means that the type of protein you eat matters! Researchers have compared animal protein–based diets with plant protein–based diets and found that gut microbes flourished from plant-based diets (with the exception of whey protein). Specifically, pea and whey protein were found to increase the good bacteria Bifidobacterium and

Lactobacillus while decreasing pathogenic bacteria in the gut.[194] More good bacteria in the gut increases short chain fatty acids, supporting digestion and calming inflammation.

Research has shown that consuming too much animal protein rather than plant-based foods harms the ratio of healthy gut microbes to pathogenic ones.[195] Promoting healthy gut microflora by including more plant-based protein will have a positive effect on the skin because gut microbes have ability to regulate immune receptors that communicate with the skin and control chronic inflammation. Further, plant proteins are natural detoxifiers because of their fiber content, which can absorb and expel endotoxins from the body before they can enter the bloodstream (and reach the skin), and provide a good source of skin-loving vitamins, minerals and antioxidants. All in all, there are many health- and skin-related reasons to increase your intake of plant-based proteins!

FATS

We know the health risks associated with the typical Western diet, which consists of too much saturated and trans fats (meats, dairy, processed foods) and not enough mono- and unsaturated fats (fish, plant-based oils, nuts, seeds). This chronic imbalance has predisposed us to many health problems and diseases. Moreover, different types of fats also affect the gut microbiota. Studies have shown that consuming a diet high in saturated fats reduces the presence of good lactic acid bacteria and causes inflammation in the gut.[196] However, diets based in mono- and unsaturated fats from high-fat fish (such as salmon) were found to increase the abundance of good bacteria and helped to control inflammation in the gut.[197] Inflammation in the gut negatively affects digestion and increases the incidence of leaky gut syndrome and inflammation

within the body, both of which can negatively impact skin's health and appearance. Moreover, healthy fats are so important for skin because they make up skin cell membranes (cell walls) that help keep your skin glowing, smooth and plump in appearance.

CARBOHYDRATES

There are two forms of carbohydrates: digestible and non-digestible. Digestible carbohydrates are degraded to their simplest form such as sucrose, glucose, fructose and lactose. Although the evidence is mixed on simple sugar's effects on the microbiota, artificial sweeteners may be more of an issue. Current evidence shows that artificial sweeteners such as saccharin, sucralose and aspartame may create microbial dysbiosis and decrease the activity of good bacteria in the gut. In this way, artificial sweeteners could be potentially more harmful than natural sugars to the microbial ecosystem.[198] If you're looking for something to sweeten your coffee or tea, try honey instead of artificial sweeteners or white sugar. Commonly used in traditional medicine, honey is regaining attention because of its strong antioxidant, pre- and probiotic, and antimicrobial properties. It has prebiotics, probiotics, zinc and antioxidants, and has the ability to target pathogenic bacteria without unsettling the good resident gut bacteria. In fact, it enhances the growth of beneficial gut microbes. When used sparingly, it's a great alternative to white sugar and artificial sweeteners! It can also be used in skincare (see Chapter 7).

Fiber and resistant starches are "non-digestible" carbohydrates, meaning they pass undigested through the small intestine and move to the large intestine where they are fermented by resident gut microorganisms. When the fiber provides a source of fuel for the microbes and modifies the intestinal environment, this is known as a *prebiotic fiber*.[199] We have discussed the effects of prebiotics for

healthy skin, and from a dietary perspective, it is their influence on immune and inflammatory markers that indirectly helps to maintain healthy, balanced skin.

Finally, eating low-glycemic foods (high-fiber whole grains, most vegetables, and beans and legumes) is not only healthier for you but also better for your skin. When you consume too many processed carbohydrates such as white breads, rice, pasta and instant cereals, these foods are quickly digested, causing "spikes" in blood sugar levels that can attack and break down skin connective tissue.

ANTIOXIDANTS—POLYPHENOLS

Free radicals are always around us, either through normal metabolic processes or from our environment, and they are in constant "check" with their counterpart, antioxidants. We're well-equipped with an antioxidant network that keeps free radicals in control. But if this network is chronically overstressed or out of balance, nutrition can provide additional sources of supportive antioxidants. Because the skin is consistently exposed to environmental aggressors from our outside environment, antioxidants play an important role for the maintenance of healthy skin.[200] Important antioxidants for the skin include vitamins A, C, E and D; and a broad group of antioxidants from carotenoids and polyphenols.[201] We cannot produce these antioxidants ourselves, so they must be obtained from our diet.

Polyphenols define a broad group of antioxidants from plants, including catechins, flavonoids, anthocyanins, proanthocyanidins and phenolic acids found in plant-based foods, seasonings, oils, teas and wine.[202] This class of antioxidants is great for skin nutrition. Polyphenols, along with another antioxidant group, carotenoids, are clinically proven to promote healthy skin when taken through

dietary or supplemental sources (grapeseed extract, resveratrol, cocoa flavanols and lycopene, to name a few). The Mediterranean diet is also dense with antioxidant polyphenols from plant-based foods, wine and oils, and has shown to have superior skin benefits over more Westernized and modern diets.[203] There is one downside to polyphenols: They're sensitive and fast-acting, meaning they can be unstable and neutralized quickly in the body. To reap their benefits, you should get them from a variety of sources and preferably several times throughout the day.

Beyond their antioxidant benefits, polyphenols also have the ability to destroy harmful pathogens and help good microbes flourish in the gut.[204] Knowing what we do about the gut-skin axis, this means polyphenols benefit our skin through the gut too. Amazing! Let's discuss this a bit more.

Polyphenols are natural pathogen fighters. The most powerful inhibitors against pathogens are found in green and black teas. Based on clinical data, the group of catechins in tea has the capacity to inhibit the growth of many pathogens such as *E. coli*, salmonella, candida, *Helicobacter pylori* and more.[205] Tea catechins also encourage the activity of healthy residential bacteria in the gut, including Bifidobacterium and Lactobacillus.[206] One study found that daily consumption of red wine polyphenols for four weeks significantly increased the number of healthy microorganisms in the gut.[207] (But remember, everything in moderation!) Anthocyanins found in red wine and most berries have been shown to encourage the growth of lactic acid bacteria, while inhibiting pathogens and gut inflammation.[208] The largest family of polyphenolic compounds, flavonoids, found in cocoa and citrus fruits, have also been shown to modify gut microbiota by affecting how bacteria adheres to intestinal cells.[209] Cruciferous vegetables including broccoli, cabbage, Brussels sprouts, arugula, bok choy, cauliflower and collard

greens contain biomolecules that modify the microbiota and control gut inflammation.[210]

So if you're thinking fruits, vegetables and polyphenol-rich foods should be on your radar, you're right! They provide antioxidants, help to destroy pathogens before they can get absorbed into the bloodstream, and, through enhancing healthy gut microbiota, help regulate and balance skin health.

WHERE TO FIND POLYPHENOLS

Based on clinical data, the following dietary sources not only provide antioxidant benefits but are also effective in promoting a balanced gut (and skin) microbiome:

* Black and green teas
* Citrus fruits
* Red wine
* Apples, berries
* Cocoa
* Soy[211]

FLOURISH WITH FERMENTED FOODS

Our ancestors have consumed fermented foods for centuries, from wine, cheese, and yogurt, to vegetables and coffee. When a food is fermented either through manmade or spontaneous methods, the chemical structure of the food is modified by microbes. This

results in a more readily digestible food that is rich in probiotics and enzymes that ease digestive stress and improve nutrient absorption.

Probiotics in fermented foods balance the microbiota, encouraging an abundance of healthy bacteria while controlling the overgrowth and activity of harmful microbes. Moreover, they have an anti-inflammatory effect, both within and on the body, and are able to modify and regulate our overall immune system. Fermented foods can also synthesize certain nutrients and metabolites, such as B vitamins, to support health.[212]

There are many ways to increase your intake of probiotic-rich fermented foods. Here are some top dietary sources.

FERMENTED BEVERAGES

Kombucha is a fermented effervescent beverage prepared with black or green tea and sugar. The microbes stimulate fermentation when they come in contact with the sugar. There are so many brands available today, but I recommend you look for brands that use honey instead of white or brown sugar.

Miso is created by using koji (a type of fungus) to ferment soybeans, barley or brown rice. When used with soybeans, miso provides a good source of phytoestrogens to support and balance hormonal skin conditions such as acne and aging skin.

Kefir is produced by fermenting a milk with kefir grains. The grains that are rich in lactic acid bacteria are removed after the fermentation process. Traditionally produced with cow's milk, kefir can also be made from goat, soy, rice, nut and coconut milks.

FERMENTED FOODS

Yogurt contains probiotics that help to break down some of the milk sugar (lactose), which is why some lactose-intolerant people can consume dairy yogurts. Look for yogurts that state "contains active cultures" and that are sourced from organic and grass-fed cow, goat or sheep milks.

Cultured vegetables such as sauerkraut and kimchi are rich in enzymes, organic acids that promote healthy gut microbes, fiber and nutrients. Kimchi is a vegetable-based Korean dish made from cabbage, ginger and garlic among other seasonings and is often eaten with rice-based meals. Note that commercial brands are not as healthy as homemade and unpasteurized versions.

Cheese can be a rich source of probiotics, but be sure to find those that are unpasteurized and have been aged for six months or more. Nut and seed cheeses are also great options and are less stressful on the digestive system.

Pickles that are real, fermented pickles should be made with cucumbers and brine (salty water). Read the label and look for "lactic-acid fermented pickles."

Tempeh is made from naturally fermenting soybeans and contains all the essential amino acids, making it a great source of protein and probiotics.

Natto is a traditional Japanese dish made from fermented soybeans, making it a rich probiotic source.[213]

You might be thinking, "what about vinegars?" Most commercial brands do not contain probiotics. However, traditionally processed or raw versions of apple cider or balsamic vinegars do contain some probiotics and other acids that support pre- and probiotic

activity in the gut. You can add 1 tablespoon to a smoothie or take with water once or twice per day to support microbial symbiosis within the gut.

MICROBE-FRIENDLY HERBS AND SPICES

Herbs and spices are often overlooked, but they are one of my favorite ways to give my meals a nourishing boost! They have strong antioxidant and antimicrobial properties that foster healthy, balanced skin. You will find many herbs and spices in natural skincare products as well because of their topical benefits. I will touch upon some of those in Chapter 7.

Herbs and spices have long been used to flavor dishes and as remedies in traditional medicine. They can be sourced from different parts of a plant, such as clove from flower bud, pepper from fruit, cinnamon from bark, or ginger from a root. They are classified by their aroma and flavor: aromatic, pungent, hot, sweet, spicy, sour, bitter and astringent. Numerous studies prove that many herbs and spices possess strong antimicrobial and antioxidant properties that combat food spoilage and treat certain ailments. Interestingly, the most powerful antimicrobial herbs and spices also have the highest concentrations of those important polyphenol antioxidants we explored earlier in this chapter.[214]

Let's take a look at some of the best herbs and spices for our microbe-friendly nutrition plan:

Clove (Eugenia caryophyllata) is widely used in antiseptic medicine and as a food additive to enhance shelf life. Clove has been tested against pathogenic microbes and compared to other herbs and spices, and has consistently outperformed the others in antimicrobial potency. Its main antimicrobial component is eugenol.

Oregano (Origanum vulgare) is commonly used in many popular dishes. The main active ingredients responsible for oregano's antimicrobial action are carvacrol and thymol.

Thyme (Thymus vulgaris) contains the major active compound thymol.

Fennel (Foeniculum vulgare) has seeds that possess strong antibacterial and antifungal effects.

Cinnamon (Cinnamomum zeylanicum) contains three active components: cinnamaldehyde, cinnamyl acetate and cinnamyl alcohol. Beyond its microbial properties, cinnamon helps to support and balance blood sugars, and has anti-inflammatory and soothing effects on digestion. I add it every morning to my coffee, cereals or smoothies to start my day.

Cumin (Cuminum cyminum) is packed with antioxidant and antimicrobial properties like cuminaldehyde, cymene and terpenoids.

Turmeric (Curcuma longa) includes curcumin as its main active component, and this powerhouse spice is loaded with antimicrobial, antioxidant and anti-inflammatory properties. Turmeric is clinically proven to benefit skin health when included in a diet, taken as a supplement or used topically.[215]

Basil (Ocimum basilicum) is a fragrant herb used especially for its antifungal properties.

Cilantro, Coriander Seeds (Coriandrum sativum) is a Mediterranean herb used in many dishes like sauces, curry powders, pickling spices or as a preservative. It has proven effective at low levels as an antibacterial, with strong action against fungus.

Rosemary (Rosmarinus officinalis) has been used not only in foods but also for traditional medicine and pharmaceuticals for its anti-microbial and antioxidant effects.

Garlic (Allium sativum) counts allicin as its main active antimi-crobial component. Try to use fresh garlic instead of powdered for stronger antibacterial activity.

Black pepper (Piper nigrum) taken as an essential oil is a strong antifungal.

Ginger (Zingiber officinale) is commonly found in our food and cosmetics these days! The key microbe-fighting compounds found in ginger include alpha-pinene, borneol, camphene and linalool, and are some of the strongest in controlling pathogen overgrowth.[216]

BIOME BOOSTERS—SMOOTHIES, JUICES, TONICS, BROTHS AND TEAS

These are the fastest and easiest way to boost, purify and replenish the body and skin:

Smoothies—Start your day off with a green smoothie, one of the easiest and quickest ways to get everything you need to get going. There are so many great ways to mix up ingredients so they not only taste great but provide you with balanced nutrition. You can see some of my smoothie recipes in Chapter 9.

Juices—You have probably heard different opinions on cleansing or juicing, but when you incorporate juices, tonics and teas into your diet, they really can revitalize you. Fresh juices are also easy on the digestive system, making nutrients easily bioavailable to the body. I often recommend them as boosters to take between meals, or replace one meal per day with juice. When juicing, choose

chlorophyll-rich and detoxifying greens such as spinach, kale or dandelion greens and pair with beets, apples, carrot and ginger. If you can't make your own, seek out a fresh juice bar or cold-pressed options and consume about 4 ounces between meals.

Tonics—I love bringing the lab to the kitchen to find ways to support an "on the go" lifestyle with nutritional boosts. My clients always say that one of their biggest challenges is finding the time to prepare nutritious meals. A quick way to get a nutritional boost during a busy day is with tonics. I like to make nutritional tonics or elixirs and use them for two to three days. Some nutrients may be lost during this time, but you still get a powerful boost of nutrients in one tiny serving. Plus, you save yourself from extra calories, sugar, chemicals and preservatives in commercially prepared versions. See page 148 for one microbe-friendly recipe I love to use.

Broth—Why not try a broth? Sometimes I find a warm broth very comforting. I often make a vegetable broth and replace my herbal teas with it for a week or so to give my body a different nutritional boost. This can be an easy way to add some microbe-friendly nutrients to purify and balance the body. See page 149 for a recipe.

Tea—Black and green teas are a great source of antioxidant polyphenols, and they support the gut and skin microbiomes. For an extra boost, you can even find teas with the herbs and spices discussed in this chapter. Here are some teas that are great for skin health:

* Green tea antioxidant polyphenols (catechins, EGCG). Clinical studies show that drinking green tea daily or taking it as a supplement results in supportive antioxidant photo-protective benefits for the skin (in conjunction with SPF use). Green tea's antioxidants help protect the skin by fighting

off damaging free radicals caused by chronic/excessive sun exposure.

* Rooibos tea contains two polyphenols that act as strong antioxidants in the body: aspalathin and nothofagin. Traditionally rooibos is used to help to clear skin congestion and blemishes.

* Ginger root tea gets its active constituents from the rhizome and root. Ginger soothes and calms the skin due to its strong anti-inflammatory properties. It also boosts blood circulation, helping oxygen and nutrients reach skin tissue.

* Kombucha tea is made from fermented black tea, so it contains both antioxidants and probiotics to support gut health and naturally detoxify the body and decongest the skin.

PRE- AND PROBIOTIC SUPPLEMENTS

In Chapter 4 we went through a detailed review of skin conditions related to the microbiome. In Chapter 5, I introduced you to pre- and probiotics and what to look for on a label. And although I encourage you to focus on dietary changes, and we'll discuss more of those recommendations in Chapter 8, you may also want to consider seeking out a high-quality pre- and probiotic based supplement to help you along the way.

Based on clinical evidence, I have compiled a list of skin concerns and the pre- and probiotics that work most effectively:

Acne-Prone Skin—Probiotics *L. acidophilus, L. bulgaricus, L. plantarum* and *B. bifidum*. Prebiotics containing 100 milligrams

of fructo-oligosaccharides (FOS) and 500 mg of galacto-oligosaccharides (GOS) have also been tested.[217]

Atopic Dermatitis/Eczema—Used either alone or in combination, probiotic bacteria *L. casei*, *L. rhamnosus*, *S. thermophilus*, *B. breve*, *L. acidophilus*, *B. infantis*, *L. bulgaricus* and prebiotic FOS are effective.[218]

Psoriasis—Probiotics *L. paracasei* and *L. pentosus* will help rebalance gut bacteria for psoriasis.[219]

Sensitive and Reactive Skin—*B. brev*, *L. paracasei* and *L. delbreuckii* probiotics along with prebiotic GOS improve skin hydration and barrier function for sensitive and reactive skin.[220]

Dandruff, Itchy Scalp—Probiotic *L. paracasei* is effective.[221] [222]

Skin Aging—The probiotic *L. johnsonii*, along with antioxidants, has been used for photo-damaged skin. *L. plantarum*, *L. acidophilus*, *L. reuteri* and *L. rhamnosus* have been effective in combating skin aging caused by environmental aggressors.[223]

Rosacea—Reestablishing balance within the gut and skin ecosystem is imperative. Probiotic cultures such as Lactobacilli and/or Bifidobacterium along with prebiotics and dietary changes could support conventional treatments.[224] Drinking high-quality green tea may help combat gut pathogen overgrowth and dysbiosis.

In summary, to start transitioning toward microbe-friendly nutrition, start thinking about eating clean. Being too clean in terms of overusing antibacterial soaps, for example, isn't a good thing for microbe balance and diversity. But in regard to diet, I'm talking about consuming foods in their most nutrient-dense forms while minimizing excess chemicals, preservatives or hormones that are

present in processed and commercialized foods. Here are some quick tips for cleaning up your diet:

Remove or limit processed foods, gluten, sugar and dairy (except lacto-fermented foods, such as yogurt and kefir) and alcohol (except red wine in moderation). Buy local, in-season and organic produce if possible. Try farm-raised, antibiotic and hormone-free animal-based meats and eggs, and remove all sources of artificial sweeteners in your diet. Drink purified water and high-quality herbal teas.

Over the next month, try to incorporate the following changes into your diet:

* Make Biome-Purifying Tonic (page 148) or Biome-Purifying and Detox Broth (page 149) and consume, according to directions, for one week to gently purify and boost the body with microbe-friendly nutrients. You can repeat for a second week as well.

* Remove high-allergen foods, especially gluten and dairy, and especially if you have acne-prone skin or psoriasis.

* Think about taking a pre- and probiotic supplement according to your skin type/condition or goal.

* Begin your day with warm water and ½ fresh-squeezed lemon.

* Try a green-based berry smoothie with pea or whey protein (pea protein is better for acne-prone skin or psoriasis).

* Start to follow the Mediterranean dietary principles summarized earlier in this chapter as a baseline, especially for lunch and dinner.

* Choose low-glycemic foods: whole grains, rice, bulgur, steel-cut oats, bran, peas, beans and leafy greens.

* For sweetener, choose honey or natural alternatives such as stevia or monk fruit over artificial sweeteners, and use in moderation.

* Consume black, green or kombucha tea daily.

* Have one serving *per meal* of fermented foods. Apple cider or balsamic vinegars count; using 1 tablespoon as a serving, you can add to salads or take just before a meal (note, if you are hyperacidic or have an ulcer, I would not recommend taking vinegars on their own).

* When cooking, use fresh, frozen or dried microbe-friendly herbs and spices suggested in this chapter.

* Consume ginger or fennel tea after meals to soothe digestion.

* Remember, gradual dietary changes and proper hydration are important in reducing digestive upset or distress. If you are sensitive to dietary changes, slow down a bit to allow your body to adapt.

In the next chapter we'll cover beautifying your skin biome from the outside with skincare and lifestyle tips. Then in Chapter 8, we will pull all components together for a nutritional, skincare and lifestyle plan that purifies, nurtures and balances your skin health from the inside and out. You're on your way to a healthier you!

CHAPTER 7

Microbe-Friendly Skincare

〰️

Your skin is the interface between you and the environment. It works as the first line of defense against what we expose it to every day. Skin microbes make up part of the skin barrier, and these bacterial colonies residing on the skin are crucial to how well it adapts and defends itself. Skin allergies and sensitivities have increased over the years due to a variety of reasons including the rising use of antibiotics and toxic chemicals in cosmetics, poor digestive health, environmental pollutants, and increasingly ultrahygienic lifestyles. These factors combined reduce the biodiversity of the skin's microbial colonies, leaving it more susceptible and reactive to the environments we expose it to.[225]

In earlier chapters, we learned about the toxic health concerns of certain topical ingredients used in personal care products. As awareness of these health concerns rises, advocacy groups and clean beauty retail chains who exclusively support brands made from naturally derived, non-abrasive and sustainable formulations

are growing as well. And with technological and manufacturing improvement, natural beauty lines and precision-focused formulations are proving competitive to traditional products. This is great! But rather than using the term "clean beauty" that we often see promoted within this sector, let's instead use the term "nontoxic" beauty and skincare.

This is where prebiotics, probiotics and synbiotics come in.

We have talked about the use of pre- and probiotics to rebuild the gut microflora and its interconnection with and effect on the skin. Now I want to shift our focus on the use of pre- and probiotics to boost healthy skin from the outside. By applying probiotics topically, we can help to replenish, diversify and balance skin microflora to promote skin's healthy function and appearance.

When this ecosystem is balanced, the skin can compete with and control pathogens and stressors. When this ecosystem is disrupted, even by the overactivity of normally healthy residential bacteria, then dysbiosis occurs, leaving skin vulnerable to accelerated aging and chronic conditions. The skin microbiome is swayed by pH, sebum content, barrier function and hydration. Oily, moist or dry skin favor certain residential bacteria over others, with dry skin areas being the most diverse microbial communities.[226]

Topically applied probiotics help to combat, protect, strengthen and calm the skin by:

* Interfering with pathogenic bacteria before they cause irritation or inflammatory reactions on the skin.

* Encouraging the growth and activity of good bacteria and balancing skin microflora.

* Balancing skin pH.

* Producing vitamins, proteins and fatty acids that help keep skin healthy.

* Strengthening skin barrier function, which helps to lock in skin moisture.

* Improving skin's defense against environmental pollutants and stressors, key factors in accelerated skin aging.

* Minimizing allergic intolerances or skin sensitivities.

* Prevention and/or complementary treatment for chronic skin conditions, including acne, atopic dermatitis, psoriasis and wound healing.[227]

With the increased interest and validation on probiotic-based skincare, brands are quickly adopting the concept of good bacteria for healthy skin. In Chapter 5, I mentioned there are some things you should look out for when choosing a product. Depending on the probiotic species, subspecies or strain, some will outperform others for their anti-inflammatory, anti-microbial, pH balancing, anti-aging and moisturizing properties.[228] In addition, the probiotic must be able to adhere to the skin to control, modify and rebalance skin microflora and health.

Since this industry is still a growing one, there are some differing opinions on how probiotics actually benefit our skin. Must the probiotics used be living and viable once they reach the shelves? Or is it the bioactive compounds that the probiotics create within the product that give an overall skin benefit? To date, the probiotic-based skincare products available tend to be either sourced from the environment, offering naturally occurring bacterial species and ingredients in their whole physical form; or cultivated, isolated and formulated in a lab in combination with other probiotic species, prebiotics or complementary ingredients to support the product's claim.

NATURAL ELEMENTS FOR THE SKIN MICROBIOME

In Chapter 3, I highlighted studies showing that urban city and hyper-hygienic lifestyles are deteriorating the diversity and colonization of our skin's "good" bacteria. Dysbiosis causes our skin to become more sensitive and susceptible to our environment and the products we apply to it. So how can we prevent this dysbiosis from occurring? Bacteria from land and sea can have a positive effect on the skin by modifying and rebalancing skin microflora and the molecules that they produce.

Mud, clay and mineral spring water therapies have been used for thousands of years and form the basis of many remedies today. Their natural composition provides unique properties that manage and treat skin conditions like acne, psoriasis and atopic dermatitis, and health ailments such as arthritis.[229] And with the skin microbiome at the forefront of new research, it's no surprise that researchers are investigating how mud therapy affects the microbes on our skin!

Natural muds contain the chemical and physical properties that can modify the composition and activity of the skin microbiome. They are dense with minerals like silver, copper, iron and zinc, which have strong antibacterial effects and can also contain their own microorganisms that can rebalance skin microflora. More interestingly, muds from varied regions of the world differ in their composition, absorptive and microbial properties, and provide distinctive benefits to the skin. For example, the high mineral content in French green clay works effectively on skin lesions and acne, while sulfur-rich mud from the Dead Sea has been shown to help with psoriasis. Keep in mind that while mud and clay may look similar, they can have different beneficial effects. Muds tend to be more hydrating, while clays work to draw out impurities,

congestion and excess oils in the skin. Thermal spring waters distilled from hot springs are also a naturally derived skincare secret. Thermal water is pure and rich in minerals and certain bacterium that help to draw out impurities, soothe, rebalance and hydrate the skin.[230]

Below are highlighted muds, clays and thermal spring waters clinically validated to benefit the skin through the microbiome.

Skin Health & Action on the Skin Microbiome[231]

	Natural Elements	Effects
Clay	Kisameet Clay (Canada)	With Actinobacteria, produces substances with antimicrobial activity. Strengthens skin barrier against environmental aggressors and clarifies the skin.
Thermal Spring Water	Thermal Water (France)	With *Aquaphilus dolomiae*, strong anti-inflammatory action and proven effective in management of atopic dermatitis. Another bacterium, *Vitreoscilla filiformis*, has been isolated and used effectively for the treatment of atopic dermatitis.
Mud	Thermal Mud, Euganean Basin (Italy)	With Cyanobacteria and diatoms, has strong antibacterial and antifungal properties. Diatoms can produce compounds that provide anti-inflammatory effects.
Mud	Thermal Mud, Sirmione (Italy)	With Pelobacter species, has strong anti-inflammatory and anti-microbial properties.
Mud	Dead Sea Mud (Israel)	Anti-inflammatory, anti-microbial properties and mineral-rich, including salt, sulfur magnesium and potassium, shown to work effectively on psoriasis, congested and blemished skin, and dehydrated aging skin.

True natural powerhouses for the skin! In their whole chemical and physical form, they can help nurture the skin's ecosystem. Other muds, including moor mud or algae-based mud, can also

help purify, balance and reestablish healthy skin. Whether you choose to check out a traditionally inspired spa mud treatment or do it at home, it may be time to rethink "clean" and get a little muck on your skin.

HONEY

Many cultures use honey in traditional medicine for skin treatments. From cleansing to remedies for rash and wound healing, honey provides unique therapeutic and healing properties. It possesses antimicrobial and antioxidant compounds and has the ability to encourage skin tissue repair and renewal.[232] Most importantly for the skin microbiome, honey has the ability to kill off a wide range of harmful pathogens without destroying the good residential bacteria on the skin.

When considering bringing honey into your skincare routine, quality is key! The quality of honey varies widely and depends on the floral source, as well as seasonal and environmental factors. For skin, manuka and kanuka honey, sourced mainly from New Zealand, are best.[233] The nutritive and microbial composition of these honeys have proven effective in clinical trials for the topical treatment of acne, atopic dermatitis, psoriasis, rosacea and wound healing. Natural honeys have also proven effective to ward off UV-induced skin stress, which is amazing considering it's a completely natural unaltered substance.[234] Whether you're applying honey topically or simply enjoying it as a part of your meals, take note to support our ecosystem and welfare of bees by choosing local, organic and sustainable agriculturally sourced honey.

FERMENTED DAIRY ON THE SKIN?

In the last few years, designer or "functional" food ingredients have made their way to the skincare and beauty counters, and this is

also true for probiotic-based topical products. Even topical yogurt masks can help the health of the skin. How? Lacto-fermented dairy undergoes a fermentation process when the sugar in dairy (lactose) is converted to lactic acid, which has several topical skin benefits. Along with the naturally present lactic acid–producing bacteria Lactobacillus and Bifidobacterium, yogurt helps to calm and rebalance the skin's health.[235] In one study, topically applied yogurt masks improved skin elasticity, water content and skin tone. They have also been used in treating acne and blemish-prone skin.[236] I like to use plain Greek yogurt and add a probiotic capsule and some honey to help clarify and nourish my skin once a week.

Here's that recipe, along with some variations I like as well. Remember to always do a skin patch test on the forearm before applying a mask to the face.

Nourishing Mask with Probiotics and Honey

1 probiotic capsule (choose a symbiotic blend of at least 10 billion CFU)

3 tablespoons plain Greek yogurt

1 tablespoon raw honey

1. In a clean glass bowl, break the probiotic capsule and mix with the yogurt and honey.

2. Avoiding the eye area, apply evenly to the face and neck.

3. Leave on for 15 to 20 minutes.

4. Wipe off *very gently* with a damp lukewarm cloth and pat dry.

5. Apply a probiotic-based moisturizer for an extra dose of nourishment.

6. Repeat once to twice per week.

✳ Probiotics provide a source of good bacteria and nurture skin microflora while combating harmful bacteria.

✳ Probiotic lactic acid bacteria gently exfoliate the skin's surface.

✳ Honey is a source of prebiotics and acts as a humectant, promoting skin moisture and providing antimicrobial properties.

TO HYDRATE AND REVITALIZE

✳ Add 1 teaspoon of grapeseed oil, avocado oil or olive oil to the Nourishing Mask.

✳ Add 5 drops of rose hip or carrot seed oil to the Nourishing Mask.

TO CLARIFY AND DETOX

Before applying the Nourishing Mask with Probiotics and Honey, try this mask to detoxify the skin:

✳ Combine 1 tablespoon green clay with 1 teaspoon jojoba oil.

✳ Apply to a clean, dry face and leave on for 10 minutes.

✳ Wipe gently with a damp lukewarm cloth and pat dry.

Wait 10 minutes before applying the Nourishing Mask.

✳ Add 3 drops lavender essential oil to the Nourishing Mask.

TO SOOTHE AND CALM

✳ Add 1 tablespoon of organic aloe vera gel and 5 drops chamomile essential oil to the Nourishing Mask.

To do a full-body treatment, try a purifying and balancing mud, algae or kelp body mask or bath soak (many products are commercially available). Apply to the skin and allow to soak for 15 minutes at least. After rinsing off the mask, apply some coconut oil to the body. Coconut oil is ultrahydrating, soothing and antimicrobial, so it helps to calm irritated, dry, itchy skin. Do a full-body treatment every two weeks.

WHAT TO LOOK FOR IN PROBIOTIC SKINCARE

It's important to note that you have a distinct combination of skin microflora and an ecosystem that has evolved with you. Therefore, a product can react differently from one person to another. You may need to try a few different products to find one that best suits your skin. I would also recommend looking for products that are more natural and organic and avoiding those with harmful ingredients like parabens and phthalates. The Environmental Working Group's Skin Deep Cosmetic Database is a great resource to check for safety of ingredients. Also, as mentioned in Chapter 5, formulating with probiotics can be a complex process due to their sensitivity and stability issues. There are questions within the industry regarding the best forms: freeze-dried, living or non-living. When researching this, it's hard to decipher which form is better because of conflicting evidence and the lack of regulatory standards around topical probiotics. As the industry matures, advances and understanding in this area will also improve.

Get to know what's in a product before you apply it to your skin.

PROBIOTICS NOW SKINCARE

Directions for Use: Avoiding eye area, dispense a small amount and gently apply onto cleansed face.

Active Ingredients: Water (Aqua), Glycerin, Lactobacillus, Olea Europaea (Olive) Fruit Oil, Vitis Vinifera (Grape) Leaf Extract, Lactobacillus/Lemon Peel Ferment Extract, Inulin, Linum Usitatissimum (Linseed) Oil, Sodium Hyaluronate, Tocopherol, Rosmarinus officinalis (Rosemary) Oil Extract

Free from: Parabens, Sulfates, Phthalates, Dyes, Gluten, Synthetic fragrance, GMOs, Triclosan, Alcohol, Dimethicone, Silicone, Animal-derived ingredients

Expiration 12/19

Water = Ingredients are listed from greatest to least amount. So those top ingredients account for higher percentages within the product.

Lactobacillus = Look for probiotic species, subspecies or specific strains. Also note where it sits on the label.

Olive = Common names of ingredients are presented next to their formal chemical names.

Lactobacillus/lemon peel = Some probiotics can be found combined with other actives as shown here with lemon peel.

Inulin = Source of prebiotics. Can be listed as a common name or derived from plant or food source with Latin and common name.

Rosimarinus officialis (rosemary) oil extract = Look for natural preservatives in the formula. Beware of some

ingredients camouflaging others. Some preservatives may be masked as fragrances. If you're unfamiliar with an ingredient, do some research or check an ingredients safety database such as the Environmental Working Group.

Free from = Check the "free from" list. The most transparent brands usually provide the most detail behind their formulations and quality standards. Watch though for masking of certain ingredients; for example, if a product states "alcohol free," make sure it is free from ethyl, cetyl, stearyl, cetearyl or lanolin alcohols.

Expiration = Check the expiration date (expiry) and storage conditions to keep product fresh.

NOTEWORTHY INGREDIENTS

When you're looking at a probiotic label, seek out a synbiotic blend of probiotic strains and prebiotics to fuel them. I have mentioned those probiotic species, subspecies and strains clinically validated to support the skin in Chapter 4, but let's recap and simplify it a little so you know what to seek out in a topical product.

Lactobacillus species—This lactic acid bacteria is the most diverse group of strains and most widely studied for its ability to stick to and benefit the skin.

Bifidobacterium species—Well-documented to work effectively with Lactobacillus for skin and offers moisturizing properties.

Vitreoscilla filiformis—Strengthens the skin barrier and calms and balances skin.

Nitrobacter—This bacterium, found in the sea and soil, is interesting because it produces nitrate, a molecule that has a beneficial

procirculatory effect within the body and on the skin. It has been found to provide antifungal properties and helps to protect skin cells from environmental aggressors.[237]

Prebiotics—Ideally you want to look for prebiotic sugars such as oligosaccharides, galacto-oligosaccharides and fructo-oligosaccharides or other food-derived prebiotics. These provide a source of fuel for the probiotics within the product and encourage your skins good bacteria to flourish.

Probiotic metabolites—Probiotics can die off and produce metabolites that may also have positive effects on the skin. In fact, skincare brands are starting to market these byproducts as active ingredients along with the probiotics! Some of these are organic acids that help to rebalance skin pH, calm and moisturize the skin, like hyaluronic acid, an enzyme that promotes the production of moisturizing ceramides, and lipoteichoic acid, which helps to strengthen the skin barrier and calm skin redness. Glycoproteins can encourage resilient and smooth skin.

Complementary ingredients—These help to strengthen and protect the skin barrier, which will support the skin microbiome. Topical products are often formulated with complementary ingredients such as phytoceramides, along with food- and botanical-based antioxidants.

PROBIOTIC BACTERIA FOR SKIN CONDITIONS

Based on clinical studies on probiotics and skin health, below are some of the most applicable ones for certain skin health conditions. You can use this as a reference when reviewing skincare labels.

Anti-Aging, Antipollution and Hydration/Glow—All Lactobacillus species including *Lactobacillus johnsonii*, *Lactobacillus plantarum*,

Lactobacillus acidophilus and *Lactobacillus rhamnosus,* as well as *Bifidobacterium breve* and *Streptococcus thermophilus* (this bacterium actually helps your skin manufacture ceramides, for a strong skin barrier and ultimate hydration).[238]

Acne and Blemished-Prone Skin—*Bacillus coagulan, Bifidobacterium bifidum, Bifidobacterium lactis, Lactobacillus acidophilus, Lactobacillus bulgaricus, Lactobacillus casei, Lactobacillus paracasei, Lactobacillus plantarum, Lactococcus lactis, Enterococcus faecalis* and *Streptococcus salivarius.*[239]

Anti-inflammatory and Sensitive Skin Conditions—*Bifidobacterium longum, Lactobacillus casei, Lactobacillus fermentum, Lactobacillus paracasei* and *Streptococcus thermophilus.*[240]

Atopic Dermatitis—*Lactobacillus casei, Lactobacillus rhamnosus, Streptococcus thermophilus, Bifidobacterium breve, Lactobacillus acidophilus, Bifidobacterium infantis, Lactobacillus bulgaricus* and *Lactobacillus salivarius.*[241]

Psoriasis—*Lactobacillus paracasei, Lactobacillus pentosus* and *Bifidobacterium infantis.*[242]

Rosacea—Lactobacilli and Bifidobacterium species.[243]

Dandruff/Itchy Scalp—*Lactobacillus paracasei.*[244]

BEAUTIFYING YOUR BIOME FROM THE OUTSIDE

Caring for the health of your skin through the microbiome is also about building and maintaining a strong skin barrier. With the compounding of factors like overcleansing, applying harsh ingredients and masking our skin with lotions, makeup and fragrances, it may be time to rethink and simplify our approach to skincare.

Plus, the environmental effects we discussed in Chapter 3 can put the skin in a more serious state of dysbiosis. From the research I have compiled throughout writing this book, I want to provide some general guidelines for microbe-friendly skincare. You may want to speak to your dermatologist or esthetician for more individualized recommendations.

Rethink your daily routine to purify, nurture and balance your skin biome.

* Use lukewarm to cooler temperatures when cleansing your face. Avoid showering or sitting in the bath too long in very hot water. Hot water strips away skin's natural oils.

* Pat your skin gently when cleansing or drying with a towel.

* Step away from using exfoliants, peels and deep cleansers too often. Although they're great to remove dead skin cells and excess debris, the continuous abrasive action breaks down the skin barrier (where those skin microbes are most active) and can make your skin more sensitive and susceptible to pollutants and products you apply.

* Switch to natural and gentle cleansers (rather than soaps) that have water as the main ingredient instead of alcohol or sulfates. Look for cleansers that may include pre- and probiotics, certified-organic ingredients, oils and micellar water, for example.

* Use a daily moisturizer with pre- and probiotics along with complementary ingredients such as phytoceramides, carotenoid and polyphenol antioxidants to nurture your skin and help your microbiome flourish.

✳ At night, go for richer moisturizers to help your skin microbiome reset itself while you sleep.

✳ For treatments, try naturally sourced face, scalp and body masks. For aging and sensitive skin, look to mud or algae-based masks for extra hydration. For oily and congested skin conditions, try a pink or green clay mask to help draw out impurities and excess oils. Using whole and naturally sourced products will not only provide microorganisms and their metabolites but also vitamins, mineral salts and antioxidants to purify and rebalance the skin. One of my favorite scalp and hair treatments is the Pink Hair and Scalp clay mask from ESPA. And now I know why it works so well! Thermal water products also provide soothing and balancing effects on the skin. Spritz daily or follow the manufacturer's directions for use.

✳ Reduce the number of cosmetics you apply to your face daily. Excess makeup exposes your skin to chemicals, smothers the skin and requires extra cleansing to wipe off. Simplify your routine or amount applied daily. Switch to mineral-based and organic brands if possible.

With everything we've learned about the skin microbiome and probiotics, why wouldn't you want to try these in your skincare? And although there are general species of bacteria that dominate and colonize on the skin, remember that your skin microbiome is unique and influenced by the lifestyle you lead and what you expose it to. So it's important to consider your current skin health status, the products you apply to it, as well as your diet and environmental exposure for balanced healthy skin. The concept of symbiosis and biodiversity moves beyond microbes colonizing on the skin; it's about coexistence on a macro level that brings it back to those microscopic microorganisms that help keep your skin healthy, clear and luminous.

Putting It Together: The Beauty Biome Lifestyle

∿

A single square centimeter of the human skin can contain up to 1 billion microorganisms. These diverse microbial communities protect us from infection but may also aggravate and increase skin sensitivity and other conditions if we don't nurture our skin and expose it to a biodiverse ecosystem.[245]

When nurtured and balanced, the skin microbiome can adapt and act as a gatekeeper between you and potentially harmful pathogens and pollutants. When out of balance, the ability for skin bacteria to control and stop pathogens and pollutants in their tracks is compromised. Your skin is left vulnerable and oversensitized to these environmental stressors. To truly nurture the skin microbiome, we need consider an integrated approach to what we consume and expose our skin to every day. As we have learned, there are multiple factors that affect our microbiome, including:

* Environmental and external factors—nutrition, prebiotics, probiotics and synbiotics; psychological stress and lifestyle; air quality/exposure from indoor, urban and rural settings; topical skincare and cosmetics; pets; medications and antibiotics.

* Internal factors—aging, genetics, immune and health status, hormonal changes.[246]

Discussing either topical skincare or diet alone in relation to the skin microbiome would only be half of the story. It is through the integration of nutrition plus skincare plus lifestyle that will best benefit our skin. Therefore, I have put together some practical guidelines and tips to help you rethink your skin health through your biome, from the inside and out.

First of all, let's highlight the skin biome philosophy based on the latest skin microbiome research we have reviewed throughout this book. I have set three fundamental components for this biome-friendly lifestyle.

PURIFY—Minimize the "toxin" load you expose yourself to every-day, from what you consume to what you apply to your skin. The goal here is move toward a healthy and non-toxic approach to skincare.

NURTURE—Rebalance and nurture your skin biome through microbe-friendly nutrition, supplementation, skincare and exposure to a biodiverse environment.

BALANCE—Establish a foundational skincare, health and lifestyle routine to maintain healthy luminous skin.

BEAUTIFY YOUR SKIN BIOME—THE PLAN

In Chapter 6 we learned there are core dietary principles that can reset and repopulate the gut with good bacteria. This good gut bacteria subsequently influences the health and function of the skin and the skin microbiome. When we utilize the gut as the "gateway" to our skin, we can modify our skin health, including hypersensitive, allergic or inflammatory conditions through pre- and probiotic-focused nutrition. Based on clinical evidence, a lacto-fermented and polyphenol-rich diet are effective for rebuilding gut barrier and microflora.

Although I don't want to use the term "clean eating," it is important to look at purifying or removing the toxin load from your diet. This will help to reduce exposure to foodborne toxins and chemicals that can stress or overburden the body. Because your skin is connected with your digestive health, when the gut is unhealthy (e.g., through leaky gut syndrome, food allergens, harmful bacteria overgrowth) it can weaken skin's immunity and normal functions. By removing high-allergen, processed and hard-to-digest foods, you allow the body to rest and rebalance from the inside out. This includes white rice, breads, pastas, dairy, refined sugar and alternative sweeteners, coffee, food colorings, flavorings and preservatives.

Note: If you're interested in finding out your personal biome status before beginning the program, there are companies that now provide gut microbiome testing via stool samples. A quick internet search will provide you with several companies that deliver the test to your home and provide dietary guidelines based on your assessment once you mail the test back. These results can be beneficial when considering the skin biome, as

you will be better informed on how to nurture your skin from the inside out. This is a new and evolving trend in personalized nutrition.

BIOME BEAUTY NUTRITION ESSENTIALS

To help re-flourish those good bacteria, incorporate the following four guidelines. After a month or so, you should be able to find a pattern that best suits your diet and lifestyle.

1. Get two or three fermented, pre- and probiotic rich foods per day. You can start slowly with one serving per day and build up from there. The following are all good choices:

* Active-culture yogurt or kefir (from dairy, almond or coconut milks)

* Probiotic-rich cheese (from dairy, nuts or seeds)

* Cultured vegetables (like sauerkraut or kimchi)

* Pickles (be sure to choose those that are lactic-acid fermented)

* Tempeh

* Natto

* Miso

* Kombucha

* Unpasteurized, unfiltered and organic apple cider vinegar (dilute serving size to a 1:1 ratio with water). This can help

with digestion when taken during meal time, but don't overdo it. Also avoid if you're hyperacidic or have an ulcer.

✳ Balsamic vinegar (use with freshly made salad dressings)

2. Consider a pre- and probiotic supplement. Check for the probiotics most suitable for your skin health goal or condition. A synbiotic blend with prebiotics at least 10 billion CFU is good.

3. Add chlorophyll to water daily (about 10 to 15 drops per day). Chlorophyll is a detoxifying powerhouse and helps to control pathogen and endotoxin overgrowth, balance pH, and encourage healthy gut microflora.[247]

4. Aim to get three or four nourishing smoothies or fresh juices per week and sip on broths and biome-friendly teas daily.

MILD SYMPTOMS WITH A CHANGE IN DIET

You may notice mild side effects when you make a change in diet. These usually occur within the first week and subside after that. They may include:

Blemishes—Your skin is an eliminative organ and it is common for blemishes to occur in the first week or so when changing diet. This should subside as your skin rebalances itself.

Digestive distress—Initial changes in diet and increasing fiber can upset the digestive system. Ensure you're getting enough fluids; opt for ginger or digestive soothing teas, and perhaps slow down on dietary changes and take it a bit slower. You will eventually get there and without the distress!

Headaches/lethargy—This can be common with a change in diet, but should not last more than a couple of days.

RESTOCK YOUR KITCHEN

To get you moving toward the beauty biome plan, restock your kitchen with these nutritious microbiome-friendly, pre- and probiotic-rich foods. If possible, choose organic, in-season or frozen, hormone- and antibiotic-free, grass-fed animal protein; and wild, low-mercury fish and shellfish. If you don't have organic produce, use a natural-based fruit and vegetable soap to clear away excess residues. If you're using produce from your garden, gently wash your herbs and veggies—those keep a bit of the healthy microbes intact. Also try to avoid gluten, soy and dairy; even if you only do it for the first month to allow the digestive system to rest and reset, you may notice improvements in your skin too.

PRODUCE

Vegetables—chicory, garlic, shallots, onions, spring onions, Jerusalem artichokes, leeks, savoy cabbage, dandelion greens, asparagus, yams, carrots, radishes, beets, cucumbers, bell peppers, shitake mushrooms, kale, collard greens, spinach, sprouts, fennel, cauliflower, broccoli, beets, arugula

Fruits—bananas, watermelon, grapefruit, berries, mangos, tomatoes, cranberries, lemons

PROTEIN

Plant protein—beans and legumes (chickpeas, kidney beans, black beans, lentils), plant protein powder (pea, whey, hemp, rice)

Animal protein—mercury-free fish (anchovies, herring, wild salmon), free-range beef, chicken, turkey, lamb, omega-3–rich eggs

CARBOHYDRATES

Bran, barley, oats, wild rice, quinoa

FATS AND OILS

Avocado, extra-virgin olive oil, sunflower oil, walnut oil, flaxseed, sesame oil)

MICROBE FRIENDLY FOODS

Lacto-fermented foods—sauerkraut, kimchi, fermented vegetables, pickles, kombucha fermented tea, unsweetened yogurt, kefir or dairy alternatives

Unsweetened almond, cashew, coconut or rice milk (choose these over higher-allergen dairy or soy milks, especially for skin suffering from acne, rosacea or psoriasis)

If tolerated, raw nuts and seeds—blanched almonds, pistachios, pecans, walnuts, nut butters, flaxseeds, chia seeds, hemp seeds, pumpkin seeds, sesame seeds and sunflower seeds

Herbs and spices—clove, oregano, thyme, fennel, cinnamon, cumin, turmeric, basil, cilantro/coriander seeds, rosemary, garlic, black pepper, ginger

Teas—high-quality green, black, rooibos, ginger root, turmeric, kombucha

Raw unpasteurized honey, cocoa, coconut, balsamic vinegar, apple cider vinegar and red wine vinegars

Fresh green juices, homemade broths, soups or tonics

START YOUR DAY BIOME-FRIENDLY AND BEAUTY-INFUSED

To get every day off on a path of skin-friendly nutrition, take these basic steps first:

* Drink ½ lemon squeezed into warm water every morning.

* Drink tea of your choice (per recommended guidelines, see pages 102–103).

* Add mint or unflavored chlorophyll to water.

* Take a probiotic supplement if you have decided to use one, and follow directions for use.

For breakfast, I love to start my day off with a smoothie because they're super convenient, energizing and are an easy way to get all of those beauty-loving nutrients, including pre- and probiotics. I recommend you test the recipes starting on 140 and modify them to your preferences, but this will at least give you the fundamentals on how you can get pre- and probiotics along with beauty-infused and energizing nutrients early in the day. Functional powders, such as prebiotic inulin or collagen, can also be added to smoothies without compromising taste. If you do consider adding a supplement powder, look for certified organic versions and use within three months after opening.

As part of a skin wellness plan, collagen is important because it makes up 30 percent of the protein in the body and constitutes about 70 percent of protein in the skin. Set within the dermis (below the outermost layer of skin), collagen is the foundation of the connective tissue that supports skin's structure (and starting point where wrinkles are formed). By adding certain protein-rich foods to your diet, you can promote a healthy skin collagen production and protect your skin from premature aging. Some top collagen-boosting foods include poultry, eggs, crab, lobster, oysters, bell peppers, sweet potato, almonds, sunflower and sesame seeds, chickpeas, kidney and soy beans, and seaweed. Add them with foods high in vitamin C (essential for collagen production) too.

For collagen supplements, I prefer a marine-based product, and you don't necessarily need to take the full dosage. Recent studies are showing skin, hair and nail health benefits with doses as low as 2,000 milligrams per day. If you're not keen on animal-sourced collagen powders, there are other ways to get its benefits either through making your own bone broth (see my recipe on 147) or seeking out plant- or botanical-based ingredients, such as gotu kola (*Centella asiatica*) seed, a powerful herb used in Eastern traditional medicine and more recently in Western medicine to promote skin collagen production. As always, do your research and check with your healthcare practitioner if you are concerned about potential contraindications of dietary supplements.

BIOME BEAUTY MEALS

I collaborated with my friend Melissa Neubart, a health advocate and graduate of the Natural Gourmet Institute, who created some amazing meal suggestions and recipes based on the biome beauty guidelines and pre- and probiotic nutrition principles. These sample meal recipes work great for lunch or dinner and will guide you toward choosing the most nutrient-dense foods for the biome beauty nutrition plan.

* Chicken breast sliced, avocado, red pepper with feta (if tolerated) on bed of spinach, baby kale drizzled with Avocado-Miso Dressing (page 143)

  Green tea

* Quinoa with Red Peppers with Lemon-Herb Vinaigrette Dressing (page 141)

  Biome-friendly tea of your choice

* Vegetarian chili with onion, kidney and black beans, chili powder and cumin

  A few fermented vegetables or 2 to 3 pickles

  Ginger-turmeric tea

* "Get Your Greens" Salad with Beets and Avocado-Miso Dressing (page 143)

  Single-serving (about ¾ cup) organic low-sugar Greek-style yogurt with drizzle of honey

  Green tea

* Curried lentil soup

  Side of greens with Avocado-Miso Dressing (page 143) or Balsamic Vinaigrette Dressing (page 145)

  Green tea

* Baked Salmon with Pesto (page 142)

  Wild rice and steamed broccoli

  Miso soup

* Kimchi Omelet Anytime of the Day (page 145)

  Side of greens with Avocado-Miso Dressing (page 143) or Balsamic Vinaigrette Dressing (page 145)

  Green tea

* Savory Roasted Chickpeas (page 144)

  Arugula and peppers with Balsamic Vinaigrette Dressing (page 145)

  Miso soup or biome-friendly tea of your choice

JUICES, BROTHS AND TEAS

Add teas and broths to your daily regimen between meals or after a heavy meal to support digestion.

To boost and replenish the body and skin, pick a couple of weekends or one week each month to make some fresh juices daily. Take them once or twice per day in the morning or between meals. When you're juicing, it's a great time to do a mud treatment at the spa or at home to reap the full benefits of nutritional and skincare cleanses combined.

WHY BONE BROTH?

It may not be for everyone, but there are some good reasons to consider adding bone broth to your diet for gut and skin health.

* Strengthens gut barrier—Bone broth is recommended for the GAPS diet, a diet used to treat autism and other conditions rooted in gut dysfunction because of the gelatin and amino acids that help to soothe intestinal lining and improve nutrient absorption.

* Rich in gelatin and protein—Bone broths contain gelatin and amino acids such as proline, essential for healthy skin connective tissue for firm, smooth skin, hair and nails.

* Supports liver detoxification—Bone broths contain the amino acid glycine, which helps support liver-detoxifying pathways.

* Source of minerals—Bone broth contains calcium, magnesium, potassium and phosphorus, all important for healthy digestion, circulation, nervous system function and bone health.

BIOME BEAUTY SKINCARE PLAN

Unlike the gut, the skin is constantly exposed to microbes from our external environment. And until recently it was believed that to keep skin healthy, we needed to lead ultra-hygienic lifestyles. Now, thanks to the advancement in understanding of the skin microbiome, we know better. Much of the clinical evidence is pointing toward rethinking how we should be caring for our skin. The following skincare guidelines were developed with your skin microbiome in mind.

Clean out your skincare or beauty cabinet. A great resource for "non-toxic beauty" is the 2010 book *No More Dirty Looks: The Truth about Your Beauty Products and the Ultimate Guide to Safe and Clean Cosmetics* by Siobhan O'Connor and Alexandra Spunt. It's worth a read and is a good introduction to the concept of non-toxic or healthy beauty. And with eco-conscious cosmetic databases available today, it's easier now than ever to dig down and learn more about the health and safety of skincare and cosmetics ingredients. You can start by removing products with harsh chemicals, preservatives and deep cleansers (such as sulfates, parabens, triclosan, artificial fragrances, polyethylene glycol, oxybenzone and formaldehyde) from your bathroom cabinet. Check your cosmetics, bodycare and haircare as well to reduce your toxic load in your skincare and cosmetics. Your skin biome will thank you!

Switch to less abrasive organic, natural and pre- and probiotic-based skincare. There are many brands out there now and some may be more suited for your skin type and health goals. A good place to start looking for healthy and non-toxic beauty brands is through retailers who also live by the same philosophy. Credo Beauty (credobeauty.com) is one retailer that has done a great job in bringing together some of the highest-quality non-toxic brands in the market. You may not want to change everything in your

current skincare routine right away, but at least start with a good pre- and probiotic-based cleanser and moisturizer suited for your skin type and condition.

BIOME-NURTURING FACE TREATMENTS

Depending on your skin's sensitivity or particular conditions you're working to improve, do these treatments weekly or biweekly.

Try a mud face mask for acne-prone or congested skin. Opt for green or pink clay-based products and mud or algae-based masks for added hydration and nourishment for the skin. Look for high-quality masks that offer more purity and fewer contaminants than some of the lower-end options.

Follow up with the Soothing and Moisturizing Probiotic Mask (with added boosters for your skin type) a couple of days after the mud or clay mask. It also works well after a medical aesthetic procedure or for itchy, flaky skin. Oats and avocado soothe and moisturize the skin. You can do the this once or twice a week.

Soothing and Moisturizing Probiotic Mask

2 tablespoons plain Greek yogurt

½ ripe avocado, mashed well

1 to 2 probiotic capsules (with Lactobacillus, Bifidobacterium and Streptococcus thermophilus)

1 teaspoon raw honey

1 tablespoon oats or oat flour for a finer consistency

1. Combine the ingredients in a clean glass bowl, breaking open the probiotic capsules to combine with the other ingredients.

2. Apply to cleansed skin and leave on for 10 to 20 minutes.

3. Gently wipe off with a damp lukewarm clean cloth and pat dry.

4. Apply a rich moisturizer (night moisturizers work well), preferably with ceramides and probiotics.

BEAUTY BIOME WHOLE-BODY CARE

For cleansers, look for ultra-gentle or "biome friendly" products without sulfates, which can put your skin's pH out of whack. Soothing ingredients like oatmeal, chamomile and lavender can cleanse without stripping away oils or drying out the skin.

For moisturizers and other topical products, look for ceramide and probiotic-based ingredients that work to nurture the skin microbiome and build up the skin barrier rather than interfering with or breaking down the skin's natural ecosystem. Look for products with coconut oil because it has microbial balancing action for the skin too,

Do sweat. From exercise to saunas, sweating creates metabolites that act as prebiotics for those skin microbes.

Clothing and laundry alert: Wearing synthetic materials may disrupt skin microbes and harbor more harmful bacteria than naturally sourced clothing like cotton, hemp or linen. Natural-based textiles have also been shown to retain more favorable bacteria when they're freshly laundered than synthetics do.[248]

Spa time! Make some time to visit the spa for a traditional mud body wrap, sauna and/or hydrotherapy session. The natural elements and microorganisms in the mud or algae will detoxify the

skin, reestablish skin microflora, and nourish and tone the skin. If you would rather do an at-home treatment, dry brush your skin, especially around the thighs and stomach to stimulate circulation and lymphatic drainage. Then apply a body mud treatment and leave on for 5 to 10 minutes before entering the bath or shower. If you're in the bath, soak in the mud bath for another 10 to 15 minutes. If you're in the shower, let the natural steam penetrate into the skin for a few minutes before washing off. You can do this. Do a mud therapy treatment for your body biweekly for best results.

Dry brushing is a good way to remove skin debris and stimulate blood flow and lymphatic drainage without stripping away the skin's natural oils. Do a quick brush before entering the shower, especially on the thighs, where fluid builds up and circulation is less active.

BIOME BEAUTY LIFESTYLE

It's in the mindset. Do you remember in Chapter 1 when I introduced you to the gut-brain-skin axis? This amazing bio- and neurocommunicative network can be influenced by our mental and emotional stress. If you want to keep your skin ecosystem healthy and balanced, then try to keep your stress levels in check. Meditation and yoga can be influential in managing your stress response and can be easily incorporated into your daily/weekly lifestyle. From a class to an app at home, mix up your yoga sessions with moksha (or hot yoga), restorative yoga or meditation classes to give your mind and body the rest and balance it needs. There are also great mind-empowering apps out there like Calm or Headspace that teach you how to settle and focus the mind, as well as how to de-stress, sleep soundly and take on the daily stresses of life.

And beauty sleep is real. It's when the mind and body (and skin) renew and revitalize for the next day. Try gentle soothing teas in the evening such as chamomile, lavender, lemon balm or passionflower. There are so many nice blends available. Magnesium is also great to help calm the nervous system and body to prepare for a quiet, restful sleep.[249]

Get outdoors as much as you can. If you can, switch your exercise routine to outside. Go for more walks with your dog, get to parks, do some gardening—anything that will help you reconnect with nature and your surroundings. As you know from Chapter 3, it helps your skin balance and build a healthy ecosystem! Just remember to wear your sunscreen.

One of the best ways to reconnect with nature is gardening. Growing your own vegetables and herbs is one way to get the most from your food through microbe-rich biodiverse soil and get you outdoors. And who better to ask about this than my former colleague and friend Mike Rohlfsen, who specializes in agriculture and biotechnology (and is an avid gardener himself).

According to Mike, here are some tips to help you build a sustainable, microbially diverse garden for your blooms, herbs and produce.

> "Just to confirm your interest in gardening, if you are a newbie, take your time, do what's easy first and what you can manage with the free time you have. Don't be too ambitious and fail simply due to the fact you bit off more than you could chew. You will be encouraged by your success, even if it's in small steps
>
> Get your soil right first! Good soil is always half the battle. You can purchase good soil or if you are lucky enough to be starting with it, even better. Always amend

your soil with good organic matter sources like well-aged composts and manures. A little bit every year keeps the microbial activity in the soil healthy and allows for healthy uptake of nutrients to the plant and other things that boost plant immunity. Organic fertilizers are also very helpful, but there is also nothing wrong with your standard fertilizer as long as it's in combination with good amounts of organic matter.

Almost everywhere in North America [United States and Canada] there are good local how-tos from your nearby agricultural extension offices or universities across a wide array of crops. Do your homework beforehand so you start with the proper soil, fertilizer, the timing of the planting and other crucial things. There are hundreds of good videos on YouTube to help get you started.

Another often-overlooked point is access to sun. There is a lot of variability by plant. Some crops need a lot of sun, while some can be constantly stressed by too much. Keep that in mind when you plan—to account for shade from trees or which direction a wall faces beside the plant (south, for example, will mean a lot of sun).

Last, for things like health and inner beauty, consider colors. Colors mean antioxidants, and in some cases you can grow some really rare ones you don't normally see at the grocery store. Mix it up! Also, these properties are often not stable, lose their potency quickly and are best consumed fresh, so when you grow them in your own garden, you get fantastic access to the properties right off the plant. Green, orange, red, purple, yellow and so on all mean different antioxidants and related nutrients. Kids love this too and it can get them excited to be more

involved in the yard. Purple string beans and potatoes, who knew? Kids love that, and you might get some free labor out of it!"

It's amazing to think that everything we do, from what we consume to what we expose our skin to, will influence the microbial communities that make up the skin microbiome. And although modern technologies and research advance, we seem to be heading toward more holistic principles in how we care for our skin.

Biome Beauty Dietary Recipes

∿

Quinoa with Red Peppers

Serves 4

1 cup quinoa

2 cups water

Lemon-Herb Vinaigrette Dressing

2 tablespoons extra-virgin olive oil

¼ teaspoon fresh minced thyme

½ teaspoon fresh minced rosemary

½ teaspoon fresh minced sage

2 teaspoons lemon zest

juice of 1 lemon

2 tablespoons chopped cilantro

½ cup diced red peppers

salt and pepper

1. Bring the quinoa and water to a boil in a medium saucepan. Then, reduce the heat, partially cover and simmer for 15 minutes, or until all the water is absorbed.

2. While the quinoa is cooking, blend the olive oil, thyme, rosemary, sage, lemon zest, lemon juice and a pinch of salt. Blend until dressing is a smooth consistency, about 45 seconds. Season with salt and pepper to taste.

3. Once the quinoa is cooked, transfer to a large bowl and mix in the lemon-herb vinaigrette, cilantro and red peppers.

Tip: To create a nutty flavor, toast your quinoa. This also helps to take away the grain's bitterness. Before adding the water, in a 2-quart pot, simply add your quinoa and warm over medium-low heat. Constantly stir the quinoa for 5 to 8 minutes. You will hear a popping sound as the quinoa begins to toast. Once toasted, add the 2 cups of water and bring to a boil. Lower to a simmer and cook for 15 minutes or until all the water is absorbed.

Baked Salmon with Pesto

Serves 2

2 salmon fillets, 4 to 6 ounces each

salt and pepper

Hemp Seed Pesto

2 cups basil, chopped

1 teaspoon salt, plus more for seasoning

½ cup hemp seeds

¼ cup extra-virgin olive oil

1½ tablespoons miso paste

1 clove garlic

2 tablespoons lemon juice

salt

1. Preheat the oven to 450°F.

2. Season the salmon with salt and pepper.

3. Place salmon, skin-side down, on a nonstick baking sheet or in a nonstick pan with an oven-proof handle.

4. Bake until salmon is cooked through, 14 to 17 minutes.

5. In a food processor, blend basil, 1 teaspoon salt and hemp seeds. Pulse for 10 to 15 seconds. Add the remaining pesto ingredients and blend to combine. Season with salt to taste.

6. Top the salmon with hemp seed pesto to serve.

Tip: If you don't have basil, you can use most bitter greens, or even carrot tops. You can also switch hemp seeds out with pine nuts, walnuts or cashews.

"Get Your Greens" Salad with Beets and Avocado-Miso Dressing

Serves 2

3 beets, peeled and chopped into 1-inch pieces

2 tablespoons olive oil

1 teaspoon salt

1 tablespoon dried oregano

1 tablespoon fresh rosemary

Avocado-Miso Dressing

1 small to medium avocado

¼ cup extra-virgin olive oil

¼ cup fresh parsley, minced

¼ cup water

¼ cup lemon juice (about 1 lemon)

5 cups salad greens (like dandelion, arugula, spinach and/or dinosaur kale)

¼ cup pumpkin seeds or hemp seeds

½ cup kimchi

3 tablespoons red or white miso

2 tablespoons chopped shallot, chopped

2 tablespoons apple cider vinegar

1 tablespoon honey

1. Preheat the oven to 400°F.

2. Toss the beets with olive oil. Add 1 teaspoon salt, oregano and rosemary. Spread on a baking sheet and bake for about 35 minutes, or until beets are tender on the inside and crispy on the outside. Allow to cool.

3. Combine all the avocado-miso dressing ingredients in a food processor and blend to combine. Refrigerate.

4. Once beets have cooled, prepare the salad. Mix the salad greens with ½ to ¾ cup dressing. Top with beets, seeds of your choice and kimchi.

Savory Roasted Chickpeas

Serves 4

1 cup dried chickpeas, soaked overnight, drained and rinsed

1 bay leaf

4 sprigs fresh thyme

¼ cup extra-virgin olive oil

2 teaspoons ground cumin

1 teaspoon smoked paprika

1 teaspoon ground fennel

1 teaspoon ground turmeric

pinch of red pepper flakes

1 tablespoon lemon juice

sea salt and black pepper

lemon

1. Combine the beans with a pinch of sea salt, bay leaf, and thyme sprigs and enough water to cover. Bring to a simmer and cook for about 2 hours, or until the chickpeas are soft. Drain the beans.

2. Preheat the oven to 350°F. Toss beans in medium bowl with the olive oil, cumin, paprika, fennel, turmeric and red pepper flakes. Sprinkle with salt and pepper.

3. Transfer beans to parchment-lined half sheet pan and roast until crispy, about 15 minutes. Finish with more sea salt and a squeeze of lemon juice.

Good Bacteria for Healthy Skin

Kimchi Omelet Anytime of the Day

Serves 1 to 2

2 eggs

1 to 2 green onions, chopped

about ¼ cup kimchi

1 tablespoon olive oil

sea salt and black pepper

arugula or pea sprouts, for topping

1. Whisk together the eggs, green onions and kimchi in a medium bowl.

2. Heat the olive oil in a medium skillet over medium heat. When hot, add the egg mixture. Add a dash of sea salt and black pepper.

3. Use a spatula to separate the egg from the sides of the pan, but let settle and cook through.

4. Once cooked through, fold over and top with arugula or pea sprouts.

Balsamic Vinaigrette Dressing

Serves 4

2 tablespoons honey

1 tablespoon Dijon mustard

1 clove garlic, chopped

¼ cup balsamic vinegar

¾ cup extra-virgin olive oil

sea salt and black pepper to taste

1. Blend all the ingredients together and refrigerate.

Grilled Salmon and Vegetables

Serves 4

4 salmon fillets, about 4 ounces each

2 tablespoons extra-virgin olive oil

1 teaspoon raw honey

¼ cup fresh basil or parsley, divided

2 red or yellow bell peppers, trimmed, halved and seeded

1 medium red onion, cut into chunks

½ teaspoon sea salt and black pepper, to taste

1 lemon, cut into 4 wedges

1. Place salmon in bowl with 1 tablespoon of the olive oil, the honey, half the basil or parsley, and a dash of salt and pepper. Let sit.

2. Preheat a grill to medium.

3. Brush the peppers and onion with the remaining 1 tablespoon olive oil and season with dash of salt and pepper.

4. Place the everything in the pan with salmon skin-side down. Turn vegetables a couple times, but leave salmon and let cook for about 10 minutes, until it starts to flake.

5. Remove from the pan, place the vegetables on serving plates, then remove the salmon skin and place the salmon on the plates. Serve with fresh lemon wedges and top with the remaining chopped basil or parsley.

Bone Broth

2 to 3 cups per day

bones of 1 whole chicken (or the carcass of a roasted chicken) or whole fish fillet bones

2 to 3 sweet bay leaves

dash of sea salt

1 tablespoon black peppercorns

any vegetable scraps (onions, carrots, celery and garlic work great)

fresh filtered water

1. In a large pot, cover the chicken bones with water and bring to a boil. Let boil for 20 minutes, and skim off the film at the top. Let cool.

2. Transfer the bones to a slow cooker and cover with water, bay leaves, salt, pepper, and vegetables of choice. Cook on medium to high for 8 to 10 hours or until the bones soften. Cool and store in the refrigerator for up to one week. Consume once or twice per day between meals.

Biome-Purifying Tonic

1 (4-inch) piece fresh turmeric or 2 teaspoons organic turmeric paste

1 (3-inch) piece fresh ginger

3 lemons, peeled

4 cups spring water or coconut water

1 teaspoon raw honey, or to taste

½ teaspoon apple cider vinegar (optional)

1. If using fresh turmeric, put it through a juicer along with the ginger and lemons.

2. Pour the fresh juice into the spring or coconut water.

3. Add the honey and turmeric paste and apple cider vinegar, if using.

4. Mix well and place in a sealed glass container.

5. Drink before meals two to three times per day in 4-ounce servings.

6. Refrigerate for up to 3 days.

Biome-Purifying and Detox Broth

If you're not using organic produce, peel or remove outer layers and wash thoroughly to reduce pesticide and chemical residues.

2 beets, peeled and halved

2 carrots, peeled

2 stalks celery

3 cloves garlic, crushed

1 red onion, cut in pieces

handful of broccoli sprouts

handful of spinach

handful of kale

dandelion greens (these can be bitter so use half amount you do of spinach and kale)

1 (2-inch) piece fresh ginger, peeled

1 (1-inch) piece fresh turmeric, peeled, or ½ teaspoon turmeric paste*

1 tablespoon ground black pepper*

½ to 1 teaspoon sea salt or dulse flakes*

1. Place all the ingredients in a large pot.

2. Fill the pot with water so all the veggies are covered. Leave room at the top of the pot.

3. Bring to a boil over high heat, then reduce the heat to a gentle boil, slightly cover and cook for about 20 minutes, until the veggies are soft.

4. Let cool, then strain broth into a glass container and seal.

5. Consume like a tea, 2 to 3 times per day. Store in the refrigerator for up to 1 week.

*You can use herbs and spices to taste and even try some others recommended in this chapter.

Fresh Juices

Choose dark greens such as spinach, baby kale and dandelion greens. Beets, apples, carrots, celery and cucumber work well to help detoxify and revitalize the body. Add a small piece of fresh ginger and turmeric too!

Luminous Skin and Antioxidant Smoothie

¾ to 1 cup coconut or almond milk

¼ cup filtered water

2 tablespoons high-protein Greek yogurt

½ scoop (or about 15 grams protein) pea, hemp or whey protein powder

½ cup fresh or frozen blueberries

handful of organic spinach leaves

1 teaspoon flaxseed oil

½ teaspoon flaxseeds or flax meal

½ teaspoon raw honey

Blend all ingredients together and serve.

BEAUTY WELLNESS FACTS

Pea protein, yogurt, honey—promote good gut bacteria

Blueberries—contain anthocyanins (antioxidant, support collagen production), good source of pectin to clear intestinal toxins

Flax—source of fiber, lignans (phytoestrogen/hormone-balancing properties) and omega-3 fatty acids for glowing skin

Clarifying Smoothie

¾ cup almond or coconut milk

¼ cup dairy or nondairy kefir

1 scoop (or about 15 grams protein) pea or hemp protein powder

½ cup frozen mixed berries

handful of spinach or baby kale leaves

¼ teaspoon ground turmeric

½ teaspoon high-quality spirulina or chlorella powder

1 teaspoon chia or hemp seeds

dash of ground cinnamon

Blend all ingredients together and serve.

BEAUTY WELLNESS FACTS

Kefir—source of probiotics for gut and skin health

Spinach and kale—contain vitamin K to balance blood sugar and magnesium to calm stress, source of skin-loving zeaxanthin

Turmeric—antioxidant, anti-inflammatory and helps to control pathogen overgrowth

Spirulina/chlorella—concentrated source of chlorophyll, phytonutrients, vitamins and minerals to purify and clear skin

Cinnamon—blood-sugar balancing effects and anti-microbial properties

Fortifying Skin, Hair and Nails Smoothie

1 cup filtered water

¼ cup nondairy kefir milk

½ scoop (or about 15 grams protein) pea, whey or hemp protein powder

½ scoop (about 2,000 milligrams) unflavored marine-collagen peptides

½ ripe avocado

½ cup fresh or frozen berries

1 teaspoon chia or hemp seeds

½ teaspoon raw honey

BEAUTY WELLNESS FACTS

Kefir and honey—source of pre- and probiotics

Protein and collagen peptides—constituents and building blocks for firm skin, healthy hair and nails

Avocado—source of antioxidant carotenoids, omega-3 fatty acids and biotin for dewy skin and sleek hair

"Glo" and Go Smoothie

½ cup nut, rice, coconut or soy milk

½ cup nondairy kefir milk

½ scoop (about 15 grams protein) protein powder

½ cup fresh or frozen raspberries

½ teaspoon cocoa powder

¼ to ½ teaspoon organic maca powder

1 teaspoon flaxseed oil

¼ to ½ teaspoon inulin powder

Blend all ingredients together and serve.

BEAUTY WELLNESS FACTS

Kefir and inulin—source of pre- and probiotics

Raspberries—excellent source of fiber, vitamin C and polyphenol antioxidants

Cocoa—source of flavanols that promote blood flow, pushing oxygen and nutrients to skin tissue

Maca—adaptogen for energy and stamina against physical and mental stress

Conclusion

∿

My microbiology classes in university influenced my preferences for certain foods, the cooking methods I use and the establishments I choose to eat in today.

However, I never would have expected to be here today writing a book about bacteria for healthy skin! Yet, after months of research and as the chapters progressed, the natural unfolding of the intricate nature and relationship we have with microbes truly fascinated me. The way they work inside our body and outside on our skin to protect and adapt to our environment to keep us healthy and balanced is remarkable.

But as urban living, toxic lifestyles and products, and ultra-hygienic routines have taken preference over more natural and diverse eco-conscious living, those good bacteria and microbes that work to keep our skin healthy are no longer present in our daily lifestyle.

With this lack of diversity, we're putting our microbiome into a state of dysbiosis, both within the body and on our skin. The skin is the most exposed and dynamic organ when it comes to the microbiome, and research is increasingly suggesting a lack of microbial diversity and/or imbalance of normally present resident bacteria as leading factors in the increasing incidence of reactive and chronic skin conditions. Sensitive skin, acne, atopic dermatitis, psoriasis, rosacea and dandruff have all been connected in clinical research with a predominance, imbalance or lack of microbial

diversity when compared to healthy skin. Moreover, these imbalances impact immune and inflammatory metabolites that further impair the skin, and taken altogether the skin becomes more susceptible to everyday environmental stressors, ingredients we apply to it and even the foods we consume.

With this advancing research, interest in pre- and probiotics has also taken predominance within the skincare industry. New studies and brands are emerging and highlighting the benefits of prebiotics, probiotics and their metabolites to help replenish and balance the skin microbiome and ecosystem for healthy luminous skin. And as this research evolves, a better understanding of precise properties and mechanisms of pre- and probiotics will allow for more specified treatments for chronic skin conditions and also help to keep our skin healthy and resilient. Along with this, more cohesive and industry-approved regulatory guidelines will improve product efficacy and make them more readily available in the market.

But skincare is only part of the story. Throughout these chapters, we have learned that it is a collective approach that includes lifestyle, nutrition, mindset and skincare to nurture and balance the skin microbiome. Simplifying our routines, getting outdoors and managing stress keep our skin ecosystem balanced and healthy.

And as I have written this book, I have kept my eye focused on the latest research to help educate and potentially simplify for you this complex and revolutionary way we can care for our skin, health and the environment in which we live. The pendulum has shifted, and we are, I believe, entering a new era in which microbes are our friends.

In health and beauty,

Paula

Notes

〜〜〜

1. Aline Rodrigues Hoffmann, "The Cutaneous Ecosystem: The Roles of the Skin Microbiome in Health and Its Association with Inflammatory Skin Conditions in Humans and Animals," *Veterinary Dermatology* 28, no. 1 (2017): 60–e15.

2. Barry Ladizinski, Riley McLean, Kachiu C. Lee and David J. Elpern, "The Human Skin Microbiome," *International Journal of Dermatology* 53, no. 9 (2014): 1177–79.

3. James A. Sanford and Richard L. Gallo, "Functions of the Skin Microbiota in Health and Disease," *Seminars in Immunology* 25, no. 5 (November 2013): 370–77.

4. J. A. Foster and K. A. McVey Neufeld, "Gut-Brain Axis: How the Microbiome Influences Anxiety and Depression," *Trends in Neuroscience* 36, no. 5 (May 2013): 305–12.

5. Petra Arck et al., "Is There a 'Gut-Brain-Skin axis'?" *Experimental Dermatology* 19, no. 5 (May 2010): 401–405.

6. Genetic Science Learning Center, "What Are Microbes?" Learn. Genetics, accessed October 2018, https://learn.genetics.utah.edu/content/microbiome/intro/.

7. Magdalena Muszer et al., "Human Microbiome: When Friend Becomes Enemy," *Archivum Immunologiae et Therapia Experamentalis* 63, no. 4 (August 2015): 287–98.

8. K. L. Baquerizo Nole, E. Yim and J. E. Keri, "Probiotics and Prebiotics in Dermatology," *Journal of the American Academy of Dermatology* 71, no. 4 (June 2014): 821–41.

9. American Psychological Association, "Stress in America: Coping with Change" (survey), 2017.

10. V. Niemeier, J. Kupfer and U. Gieler, "Acne Vulgaris—Psychosomatic Aspects," *Journal of the German Society of Dermatology* 4, no. 12, (December 2006): 1027–36.

11. Shadi Zari and Dana Alrahmani, "The Association Between Stress and Acne Among Female Medical Students in Jeddah, Saudi Arabia," *Clinical, Cosmetic and Investigational Dermatology* 10 (2017): 503–506.

12. W. Bowe, N. B. Patel and A. C. Logan, "Acne Vulgaris, Probiotics and the Gut-Brain-Skin Axis: From Anecdote to Translational Medicine," *Beneficial Microbes* 71, no. 4 (October 2014): 185–99.

13. Zari et al., "The Association Between Stress and Acne Among Female Medical Students in Jeddah, Saudi Arabia," 503–506. Bow et al., "Acne Vulgaris, Probiotics and the Gut-Brain-Skin Axis: 185–99.

14. Petra C. Arck et al., "Neuroimmunology of Stress: Skin Takes Center Stage," *Journal of Investigative Dermatology* 126, no. 8 (August 2006): 1697–1704; Pierre-Yves Morvan and Romuald Vallee, "Evaluation of the Effects of Stressful Life on Human Skin Microbiota," *Applied Microbiology Open Access* 4, no. 1 (2018).

15. Alexander Panossian and Georg Wikman, "Effects of Adaptogens on the Central Nervous System and the Molecular Mechanisms Associated with Their Stress—Protective Activity," *Pharmaceuticals* 3, no. 1 (January 2010): 188–224.

16. Laura S. Weyrich et al., "The Skin Microbiome: Associations Between Altered Microbial Communities and Disease," *Australasian Journal of Dermatology* 56, no. 4 (November 2015): 268–74.

17. Barry Ladizinski et al., "The Human Skin Microbiome." *International Journal of Dermatology* 53, No. 9, (September 2014): 1177–79.

18. Shenara Musthaq, Anna Mazuy and Jeannette Jakus, "The Microbiome in Dermatology," *Clinics in Dermatology* 36, no. 3 (May-June 2018): 390–98; B. Dréno et al., "Microbiome in Healthy skin, update for dermatologists," *Journal of the European Academy of Dermatology and Venereology* 30, no. 12 (December 2016): 2038–47.

19. Zohra Zaidi and S. W. Lanigan, "Skin: Structure and Function," *Dermatology in Clinical Practice* (2010): 1–15.

20. Dréno et al., "Microbiome in Healthy Skin, Update for Dermatologists," 2038–047; Zaidi et al., "Skin," 1–15.

21. Zaidi et al., "Skin," 1–15.

22. Jef Askt, "Microbes of the Skin," *The Scientist*, accessed October 25, 2018, https://www.the-scientist.com/news-analysis/microbes-of-the-skin-37335.

23. Elizabeth A. Grice and Julia A. Segre, "The Skin Microbiome," *Nature Reviews Microbiology* 9, no. 4 (April 2011): 244–53.

24. Askt, "Microbes of the Skin"; Grice et al., "The Skin Microbiome," 244; Rodrigues Hoffmann, "The Cutaneous Ecosystem," 60–e15.

25. Rodrigues Hoffmann, "The Cutaneous Ecosystem," 60–e15.

26. Elizabeth A. Grice et al., "Topographical and Temporal Diversity of the Human Skin Microbiome," *Science* 324, no. 5931 (May 2009), 1190–92.

27. Dréno et al., "Microbiome in Healthy Skin, Update for Dermatologists," 2038–47; Rodrigues Hoffmann, "The Cutaneous Ecosystem," 60–e15.

28. Musthaq et al., "The Microbiome in Dermatology," 390–98; Dréno et al., "Microbiome in Healthy Skin, Update for Dermatologists," 2038–47; Rodrigues Hoffmann, "The Cutaneous Ecosystem," 60–e15.

29. Ladizinski et al., "The Human Skin Microbiome," 1177–79.

30. Musthaq et al., "The Microbiome in Dermatology," 390–98.

31. Scharschmidt et al., "What Lives on Our Skin," 83–89; Michael Brandwein, Doron Steinberg and Shiri Meshner, "Microbial Biofilms and the Human Skin Microbiome," *Biofilms and Microbiomes* 2, no. 3 (2016): 1–6.

32. Ibid.

33. Ibid.

34. Brandwein et al., "Microbial Biofilms and the Human Skin Microbiome," 1–6; H. H. Kong et al., "Temporal Shifts in the Skin Microbiome Associated with Disease Flares and Treatment in Children with Atopic Dermatitis," *Genome Research* 22, no. 5 (May 2012): 850–59.

35. Weyrich et al., "The Skin Microbiome," 268–74.

36. Ibid.

37. Kong et al., "Temporal Shifts in the Skin Microbiome Associated with Disease Flares and Treatment in Children with Atopic Dermatitis, 850–59.

38. Weyrich et al., "The Skin Microbiome," 268–74; Kong et al., "Temporal Shifts in the Skin Microbiome Associated with Disease Flares and Treatment in Children with Atopic Dermatitis, 850–59.

39. Weyrich et al., "The Skin Microbiome," 268–74.

40. A. Fahlén et al., "Comparison of Bacterial Microbiota in Skin Biopsies from Normal and Psoriatic Skin," *Archives of Dermatological Research* 304, no. 1 (January 2012): 15–22.

41. A. Statnikov et al., "Microbiomic Signatures of Psoriasis: Feasibility andd Methodology Comparison," *Scientific Reports* 3 (2013): 2620.

42. Fahlén et al., "Comparison of Bacterial Microbiota in Skin Biopsies from Normal and Psoriatic Skin," 15–22; Statnikov et al., "Microbiomic Signatures of Psoriasis," 2620.

43. Ladizinski et al., "The Human Skin Microbiome," 1177–79.

44. E. A. Eady and A. M. Layton, "A Distinct Acne Microbiome: Fact or Fiction?" *Journal of Investigative Dermatology* 133, no. 6 (September 2013): 2294–95.

45. Zhijue Xu et al., "Dandruff Is Associated with the Conjoined Interactions Between Host and Microorganisms," *Scientific Reports* 6 (May 2016), accessed October 25, 2018, www.nature.com/scientificreports.

46. Sophie Seite and Laurent Misery, "Skin Sensitivity and Skin Microbiota: Is There a Link?" Experimental Dermatology 27, no. 9 (May 2018): 1061–64.

47. C. P. Wild, "Complementing the Genome with an 'Exposome': The Outstanding Challenge of Environmental Exposure Measurement in Molecular Epidemiology," *Cancer Epidemiology, Biomarkers and Prevention* 14, no. 8 (August 2005): 1847–50.

48. Jean Krutmann et al., "The Skin Aging Exposome," *Journal of Dermatological Science* 85, no. 3 (March 2017): 152–61.

49. Ibid.

50. Ibid.

51. Daniel Whitby, "5 Skincare Claims on the Horizon," *Global Cosmetic Industry,* November 9, 2018, accessed November 14, 2018, https://www.gcimagazine.com/marketstrends/segments/skincare/5-Skin-Care-Claims-on-the-Horizon-500139762.html.

52. Susan L. Prescott et al., "The Skin Microbiome: Impact of Modern Environments on Skin Ecology, Barrier Integrity and Systemic Immune Programming," *World Allergy Organization Journal* 10, no. 1 (August 2017): 1–16.

53. A. Parajuli et al., "Urbanization Reduces Transfer of Diverse Environmental Microbiota Indoors," *Frontiers in Microbiology* 9, no. 84 (2018): 1–13.

54. Prescott et al., "The Skin Microbiome," 1–16.

55. Parajuli et al., "Urbanization Reduces Transfer of Diverse Environmental Microbiota Indoors," 1–13.

56. T. Haahtela et al., "The Biodiversity Hypothesis and Allergic Disease: World Allergy Organization Position Statement," *World Allergy Organization Journal* 6, no. 1 (2013): 1–18.

57. Prescott et al., "The Skin Microbiome," 1–16; Parajuli et al., "Urbanization Reduces Transfer of Diverse Environmental Microbiota Indoors," 1–13.

58. Prescott et al., "The Skin Microbiome," 1–16.

59. Pauline Trinh, Jesse R. Zaneveld, Sarah Safranek and Peter M. Rabinowitz, "One Health Relationships Between Human, Animal, and Environmental Microbiomes: A Mini-Review," *Frontiers in Public Health* 6, no. 235 (August 2018).

60. G. J. Fisher et al., "Pathophysiology of Premature Skin Aging Induced ny Ultraviolet Light," *New England Journal of Medicine* 337, no. 20 (November 2018): 1419–28.

61. Mary E. Logue and Barret J. Zlotoff, "Reflections on Smart Phones, Tablets and Ultraviolet (UV) Light: Should We Worry?" *Journal of the American Academy of Dermatology* 73, no. 3 (2015): 526–28.

62. R. S. Chapman et al., "Solar Ultraviolet Radiation and the Risk of Infectious Disease: Summary of a Workshop," *Photchemistry and Photobiology* 61, no. 3 (March 1995): 61, 223–47.

63. L. J. Rothschild, "The Influence of UV Radiation on Protist an Evolution," *Journal of Eukaryotic Microbiology* 46, no. 5 (September-October 1999): 548–55.

64. Patra Vijay Kumar, Scott N. Byrne and Peter Wolf, "The Skin Microbiome: Is It Affected by UV-induced Immune Suppression?" *Frontiers Microbiology* 10, no. 7 (August 2016): 1235.

65. Katarzyna Adamczyk, Agnieszka A. Garncarczyk and Paweł P. Antończak, "The Microbiome of the Skin." *Dermatology Review/ Przegląd Dermatologiczny* 105 (2018): 285–97.

66. Eleni Drakaki, Clio Dessinioti and Christina V. Antoniou, "Air Pollution and the Skin." *Frontiers in Environmental Science* 2 (May 2014): 1–8.

67. Janet Raloff, "Air Pollutants Enter Body Through Skin," *Science News,* October 15, 2015, accessed November 7, 2018, https://www.sciencenews.org/article/air-pollutants-enter-body-through-skin; Hye-Jin Kim et al., "Fragile Skin Microbiomes in Megacities Are Assembled by a Predominantly Niche-Based Process," *Science Advances* 4, no. 3 (March 2018).

68. T. Y. Wong, "Smog Induces Oxidative Stress and Microbiota Disruption," *Journal of Food and Drug Analysis* 25, no. 2 (April 2017): 235–44.

69. S. E. Mancebo and S. Q. Wang. "Recognizing the Impact of Ambient Air Pollution on Skin Health," *Journal of the European Academy of Dermatology and Venereology* 29, no. 12 (December 2015): 2326–32; Q. C. He et al., "Effects of

Environmentally Realistic Levels of Ozone on Stratum Corneum Function," *International Journal of Cosmetic Science* 28, no. 5, 235–44 (October 2006): 349–57.

70. Wong, "Smog Induces Oxidative Stress and Microbiota Disruption," 235–44.

71. G. Valacchi, E. Porada and B. H. Rowe, "Ambient Ozone and Bacterium Streptococcus: A Link Between Cellulitis and Pharyngitis," *International Journal of Occupational Medicine and Environmental Health* 28, no. 4 (2015): 771–74; J. Krutmann et al., "Pollution and Acne: Is There a Link?" *Clinical, Cosmetic and Investigative Dermatology* 19, no. 10 (May 2017): 199–204.

72. G. Valacchi G et al, "Ambient Ozone and Bacterium Streptococcus," 771–74; Krutmann et al., "Pollution and Acne?" 199–204; Jadwiga Rembiesa, Tautgirdas Ruzgas, Johan Engblom and Anna Holefors, "The Impact of Pollution on Skin and Proper Efficacy Testing for Anti-Pollution Claims," *Cosmetics* 5, no. 4 (2018).

73. R. Vandergrift et al., "Cleanliness in Context: Reconciling Hygiene with a Modern Microbial Perspective," *Microbiome* 5, no. 76 (July 2017): 1–12; G. Kampf and A. Kramer, "Epidemiologic Background of Hand Hygiene and Evaluation of the Most Important Agents For Scrubs And Rubs," *Clinical Microbiology Review* 17, no. 4 (October 2004): 863–93.

74. Vandergrift et al., "Cleanliness in Context," 1–12.

75. World Health Organization, "Hand Hygiene Why, How and When?" accessed November 20, 2018, http://www.who.int/gpsc/5may/Hand_Hygiene_Why_How_and_When_Brochure.pdf.

76. Ibid.

77. H. Lambers et al., "Natural Skin Surface Ph Is on Average Below 5, Which Is Beneficial for Its Resident Flora," *International Journal of Cosmetic Science* 28, no. 5 (October 2006): 359–70.

78. Ibid.

79. Ibid.

80. Ibid.

81. Adam J. San Miguel et al., "Topical Antimicrobial Treatments Can Elicit Shifts to Resident Skin Bacterial Communities and Reduce Colonization by Staphylococcus aureus Competitors," *Antimicrobial Agents and Chemotherapy* 61, no. 9 (August 2017).

82. Vandergrift et al., "Cleanliness in Context," 1–12.

83. S. R. Abeles, "Microbial Diversity in Individuals and Their Household Contacts Following Typical Antibiotic Courses," *Microbiome* 4, no. 1 (July 2016): 39.

84. Ch. Lalitha and P. V. V. Prasada Rao, "Impact of Superficial Blends on Skin Micro Biota," *International Journal of Current Pharmaceutical Research* 5, no. 3 (2013): 61–65.

85. Environmental Working Group, "Exposures Add Up Survey Results," accessed November 23, 2018. https://www.ewg.org/skindeep/2004/06/15/exposures-add-up-survey-results

86. Ibid.

87. Lalitha et al., "Impact of Superficial Blends on Skin Micro Biota," 61–65.

88. Ibid.

89. David Suzuki Foundation, "Dirty Dozen Cosmetic Chemicals." Accessed November 25, 2018.

90. Mohammad Asif Sherwani, Saba Tufail, Anum Fatima Muzaffar and Nabiha Yusuf. "The Skin Microbiome and Immune System: Potential Target for Chemoprevention?" *Photodermatology, Photoimmunology and Photomedicine* 34, no.1 (January 2018): 25–34.

91. J. Benyacoub et al., "Immune Modulation Property of Lactobacillus paracasei NCC2461 (ST11) Strain and Impact on Skin Defences," *Beneficial Microbes* 5, no. 2 (June 2014): 129–36.

92. Sherwani et al., "The Skin Microbiome and Immune System: Potential Target for Chemoprevention?" 25–34.

93. Benyacoub et al., "Immune Modulation Property of Lactobacillus paracasei NCC2461 (ST11) Strain and Impact on Skin Defences," 129–136.

94. Sherwani et al., "The Skin Microbiome and Immune System: Potential Target for Chemoprevention?" 25–34; R. D. Whitehead et al., "You Are What You Eat: Within-Subject Increases in Fruit And Vegetable Consumption Confer Beneficial Skin-Color Changes," *PLoS One* 7, no. 3(2012): e32988.

95. Vanessa Fuchs-Tarlovsky, Maria Fernanda Marquez-Barba, Krishnan Sriram, "Probiotics in dermatologic practice," *Nutrition* 32 (2016): 289–95.

96. Mary-Margaret Kober and Whitney P. Bowe, "The Effect of Probiotics on Immune Regulation, Acne and Photoaging," *International Journal of Women's Dermatology* 1, no. 2 (April 2015): 85–89; S. Parvez, K. A. Malik, S. Ah Kang and H. Y. Kim, "Probiotics and Their Fermented Food Products Are Beneficial for Health," *Journal of Applied Microbiology* 100, no. 6 (June 2006): 1171–85.

97. Parvez et al., "Probiotics and Their Fermented Food Products Are Beneficial for Health," 1171–85.

98. Mia Maguire and Greg Maguire. "The Role of Microbiota, and Probiotics and Prebiotics in Skin Health," *Archives in Dermatology Research* 309, no. 6 (August 2017): 411–21.

99. Kober et al., "The Effect of Probiotics on Immune Regulation, Acne and Photoaging," 85–89.

100. Mary Ellen Sanders. "Probiotics: Definition, Sources, Selection and Uses," *Clinical Infectious Diseases* 46, Suppl. 2 (February 2008): S58–61.

101. Parvez et al., "Probiotics and Their Fermented Food Products Are Beneficial for Health," 1171–85.

102. Vanessa Fuchs-Tarlovsky, Maria Fernanda Marquez-Barba, and Krishnan Sriram, "Probiotics in Dermatologic Practice," *Nutrition* 32, no. 3 (March 2016): 289–95.

103. Stephanie Collins and Gregor Reid, "Distant Site Effects of Ingested Prebiotics," *Nutrients* 8, no. 9 (September 2016): 1–20.

104. A. Florowska, K. Krygier, T. Florowski and E. Dluzewska, "Prebiotics as Functional Food Ingredients Preventing Diet-Related Diseases," *Food and Function* 7, no. 5 (May 2016): 2147–55.

105. Pragnesh J. Patel, Shailesh K. Singh, Siddak Panaich, and Lavoisier Cardozo, "The Aging Gut and the Role of Prebiotics, Probiotics and Synbiotics: A Review," *Journal of Clinical Gerontology and Geriatrics* 5, no. 1 (March 2014): 3-6;

106. Kavita R. Pandy, Suresh R. Naik and and Babu V. Vakil, "Probiotics, Prebiotics and Synbiotics—A Review," *Journal of Food Science and Technology* 52, no. 12 (2015): 7577–87.

107. B. Dréno et al., "The Influence of Exposome on Acne," *Journal of the European Academy of Dermatology and Venereology* 32, no. 5 (May 2018): 812–19.

108. Kober et al., "The Effect of Probiotics on Immune Regulation, Acne and Photoaging," 85–89.

109. B. Dréno et al., "Cutibacterium acnes (Propionibacterium acnes) and Acne vulgaris: A Brief Look at the Latest Updates," *Journal of the European Academy of Dermatology and Venereology* 32, Suppl. 2 (June 2018): 5–14.

110. B. Dréno et al., "Cutibacterium acnes (Propionibacterium acnes) and Acne vulgaris," 5–14; B. Dréno et al., "The Influence of Exposome on Acne," 812–819. B. Dréno et al., "Cutibacterium acnes (Propionibacterium acnes) and Acne vulgaris," 5–14.

111. Kober et al., "The Effect of Probiotics on Immune Regulation, Acne and Photoaging," 85–89; B. Dréno et al., "Cutibacterium acnes (Propionibacterium acnes) and Acne vulgaris," 5–14.

112. L. A., Volkova, I. L. Khalif and I. N. Kabanova, "Impact of the Impaired Intestinal Microflora on the Course of Acne Vulgaris," *Klinicheskaia Medistina* 79, no. 6 (2001): 39–41.

113. J. Kim et al., "Dietary Effect of Lactoferrinenriched Fermented Milk on Skin Surface Lipid and Clinical Improvement of Acne Vulgaris," *Nutrition* 26, no. 9 (2010): 902–909; Feriel Hacini-Rachinel et al., "Oral Probiotic Control Skin Inflammation by Acting on Both Effector and Regulatory T Cells," *PLoS One* 4, no. 3 (2009): 4903–11.

114. M. R. Roudsari, R. Karimi, S. Sohrabvandi and A. M. Mortazavian, "Health Effects of Probiotics on the Skin," *Critical Reviews in Food Science and Nutrition* 55, no. 9 (2015): 1219–40.

115. G. W. Jung, J. E. Tse, I. Guihua and J. Rao, "Prospective, Randomized, Open-Label Trial Comparing the Safety, Efficacy, and Tolerability of an Acne Treatment Regimen with and without a Probiotic Supplement and Minocycline in Subjects with Mild to Moderate Acne," *Journal of Cutaneous Medical Surgery* 17, no. 2 (March-April 2013): 114–22.

116. Roudsari et al., "Health Effects of Probiotics on the Skin," 1219–40.

117. F. Dall'Oglio, M. Milani and G. Micali, "Effects of Oral Supplementation with FOS and GOS Prebiotics in Women with Adult Acne: The 'S.O. Sweet' Study: A Proof-Of-Concept Pilot Trial," *Clinical Cosmetic Investigative Dermatology* (October 2018): 445–49.

118. B. S. Kang et al., "Antimicrobial Activity of Enterocins from Enterococcus Faecalis SL-5 Against Propionibacterium Acnes, the Causative Agent in Acne Vulgaris, and Its Therapeutic Effect," *Journal of Microbiology* 47, no. 1 (February 2010): 101–109.

119. W. P. Bowe, "Probiotics in Acne and Rosacea," *Cutis* 92, no. 1 (July 2013):6–7.

120. Kang et al., "Antimicrobial Activity of Enterocins from Enterococcus Faecalis SL-5 Against Propionibacterium Acnes, the Causative Agent in Acne Vulgaris, and Its Therapeutic Effect,"101–109.

121. L. Di Marzio et al., "Increase of Skinceramide Levels in Aged Subjects Following a Short-Term Topical Application of Bacterial Sphinomyelinase from Streptococcus Thermophilus," *International Journal of Immunopathology and Pharmacology* 21, no. 1 (January-March 2008):137–43.

122. Celine Cosseau et al., "The Commensal Streptococcus Salivarius K12 Downregulates the Innate Immune Responses of Human Epithelial Cells and Promotes Host-Microbe Homeostasis," *Infection and Immunity* 76, no. 9 (September 2008): 4163–75.

123. Sanders, "Probiotics," 58–61.

124. Kong et al., "Temporal Shifts in the Skin Microbiome Associated with Disease Flares and Treatment in Children with Atopic Dermatitis, 850–59; C. W. Lynde et al., "The Skin Microbiome in Atopic Dermatitis and Its Relationship to Emollients," *Journal of Cutaneous Medical Surgery* 20, no. 1 (January 2016): 21–28.

125. R. D. Bjerre et al., "The Role of the Skin Microbiome in Atopic Dermatitis: A Systematic Review," *British Journal of Dermatology* 177, no. 5 (November 2017): 1272–78.

126. Bjerre et al., "The Role of the Skin Microbiome in Atopic Dermatitis," 1272–78.

127. Kong et al., "Temporal Shifts in the Skin Microbiome Associated with Disease Flares and Treatment in Children with Atopic Dermatitis, 850–59; Lynde et al., "The Skin Microbiome in Atopic Dermatitis and Its Relationship to Emollients," 21–28; Bjerre et al., "The Role of the Skin Microbiome in Atopic Dermatitis," 1272–78.

128. Lynde et al., "The Skin Microbiome in Atopic Dermatitis and Its Relationship to Emollients," 21–28.

129. Bjerre et al., "The Role of the Skin Microbiome in Atopic Dermatitis," 1272–78.

130. Roudsari et al., "Health Effects of Probiotics on the Skin," 1219–40.

131. Bjerre RD, Bandier J, Skov L, Engstrand L, Johansen JD, "The role of the skin microbiome in atopic dermatitis: a systematic review," 1272-1278.

132. A. Balato et al., "Human Microbiome: Composition and Role in Inflammatory Skin Diseases," *Archivum Immunologiae et Therapiae Experimentalis* 67, no. 1 (February 2018): 1–18.

133. Balato et al., "Human Microbiome: Composition and Role in Inflammatory SkinDiseases," 1–18; E. A. Langan et al., "The Role of the Microbiome in Psoriasis: Moving from Disease Description to Treatment Selection?" *British Journal of Dermatology* 178, no. 5 (May 2018):1020–27.

134. Langan et al., "The Role of the Microbiome in Psoriasis?" 1020–27.

135. Farida Benhadou, Dillon Mintoff, Benjamin Schnebert and Hok Bing Thio, "Psoriasis and Microbiota: A Systematic Review," *Diseases* 6, no. 2 (June 2018): 47.

136. Benhadou et al., "Psoriasis and Microbiota," 47.

137. G. Michaëlsson et al., "Psoriasis Patients with Antibodies to Gliadin Can Be Improved by a Gluten-Free Diet," *British Journal of Dermatology* 142, no. 1 (2000): 44–51.

138. Seite et al., "Skin sensitivity and Skin Microbiota," 1061–64.

139. Mitsuyoshi Kano et al., "Consecutive Intake of Fermented Milk Containing Bifidobacterium breve Strain Yakult and Galacto-oligosaccharides Benefits Skin Condition in Healthy Adult Women," *Bioscience Microbiota Food Health* 32, no. 1 (2013): 33–39.

140. Xu et al., "Dandruff Is Associated with the Conjoined Interactions Between Host and Microorganisms."

141. M. Egert, R. Simmering and C. U. Riedel, "The Association of the Skin Microbiota with Health, Immunity, and Disease," *Clinical Pharmacology and Therapeutics* 102, no. 1 (July 2017): 62–69.

142. Egert et al., "The Association of the Skin Microbiota with Health, Immunity, and Disease," 62–69.

143. R. Saxena et al., "Comparison of Healthy and Dandruff Scalp Microbiome Reveals the Role of Commensals in Scalp Health," *Front Cell Infectious Microbiology* 4, no. 8 (October 2018).

144. P. Reygagne et al., "The Positive Benefit of Lactobacillus Paracasei NCC2461 ST11 in Healthy Volunteers with Moderate to Severe Dandruff," *Beneficial Microbes* 8, no. 5 (October 2017): 671–80.

145. P. Reygagne et al., "The Positive Benefit of Lactobacillus Paracasei NCC2461 ST11 in Healthy Volunteers with Moderate to Severe Dandruff," *Beneficial Microbes* 8, no. 5 (October 2017): 671–80.

146. A. Kammeyer and R. M. Luiten, "Oxidation Events and Skin Aging," *Ageing Research Reviews* 21 (May 2015):16–29; Adrián D. Friedrich, Mariela L. Paz, Juliana Leoni and Daniel H. González Maglio, "Message in a Bottle: Dialog between Intestine and Skin Modulated by Probiotics," *International Journal of Molecular Science* 18, no. 6 (June 2017): E1067.

147. Patra et al., "The Skin Microbiome," 1235.

148. Maguire et al., "The Role of Microbiota, and Probiotics and Prebiotics in Skin Health," 411–21.

149. D. Bouilly-Gauthier et al., "Clinical Evidence of Benefits of a Dietary Supplement Containing Probiotic and Carotenoids on Ultraviolet-Induced Skin Damage," *British Journal of Dermatology* 163, no. 3 (September 2010): 536–43.

150. Dong Eun Lee et al., "Clinical Evidence of Effects of Lactobacillus Plantarum HY7714 on Skin Aging: A Randomized, Double Blind, Placebo-Controlled Study," *Journal of Microbiology Biotechnology* 25, no. 12 (December 2015): 2160–2168.

151. A. R. Im, B. Lee, D. J. Kang and S. Chae, "Skin Moisturizing and Antiphotodamage Effects of Tyndallized Lactobacillus acidophilus IDCC 3302," *Journal of Medicinal Food* 21, no. 10 (October 2018): 1016–23.

152. S. Ní Raghallaigh et al., "The Fatty Acid Profile of the Skin Surface Lipid Layer in Papulopustular Rosacea," *British Journal of Dermatology* 166, no. 2 (February 2012): 279–87.

153. Grice et al., "Topographical and Temporal Diversity of the Human Skin Microbiome," 1190–92; Maguire et al., "The Role of Microbiota, and Probiotics and Prebiotics in Skin Health," 411–21.

154. Cesare Cremon, Maria Raffaella Barbaro, Marco Ventura and Giovanni Barbara, "Pre- and probiotic overview," *Current Opinion in Pharmacology* 43 (December 2018): 87–92.

155. Cremon et al., "Pre- and Probiotic Overview," 87-92; Joseph Pizzorno and Michael Murray, *Textbook of Natural Medicine*, 4th ed. (St. Louis, MI: Churchill Livingstone, 2013) 979–94.

156. Parvez et al., "Probiotics and Their Fermented Food Products Are Beneficial for Health," 1171–85.

157. Roudsari et al., "Health Effects of Probiotics on the Skin," 1219–40.

158. Ibid.

159. Claudio de Simone, "The Unregulated Probiotic Market," *Clinical Gastroenterology and Hepatology* 17, no. 5 (March 2018): 809–17.

160. Dragana Skokovic-Sunjic, "Clinical Guide to Probiotics in Canada," 2018 ed, accessed January 2019, https://4cau4jsaler1zglkq3wnmje1-wpengine.netdna-ssl.com/wp-content/uploads/2018/04/Clinical-Guide-Canada-2018.pdf.

161. Mandal S, Hati S. "Microencapsulation of Bacterial Cells by Emulsion Technique for Probiotic Application," *Methods Mol Biol.*1479 (2017): 273–79.

162. S. Mandal and S. Hati, "Microencapsulation of Bacterial Cells by Emulsion Technique for Probiotic Application," *Methods in Molecular Biology* 1479 (2017): 273–79.

163. J. Bucka-Kolendo and B Sokołowska, "Lactic Acid Bacteria Stress Response to Preservation Processes in the Beverage and Juice Industry," *Acta Biochimica Polonica* 64, no. 3 (2017): 459–64.

164. Gilberto Vincius de Melo Pereira et al., "How to Select a Probiotic? A Review and Update of Methods and Criteria," *Biotechnology Advances* 36, no. 8 (December 2018): 2060–76.

165. Roudsari et al., "Health Effects of Probiotics on the Skin," 1219–40.

166. U.S. Food and Drug Administration, "Policy Regarding Quantitative Labeling of Dietary Supplements Containing Live Microbials: Guidance for Industry," September 2018, accessed January 2019, https://www.fda.gov/downloads/Food/GuidanceRegulation/GuidanceDocumentsRegulatoryInformation/UCM619529.pdf accessed.

167. International Scientific Association of Probiotics and Prebiotics, "Probiotic Checklist: Making a Smart Selection," 2018, accessed January 2019, https://4cau4jsaler1zglkq3wnmje1-wpengine.netdna-ssl.com/wp-content/uploads/2018/10/Probiotic-Checklist-Infographic.pdf.

168. GianMarco Giorgetti et al., "Interactions Between Innate Immunity, Microbiota, and Probiotics," *Journal of Immunology Research* 2015: 501361.

169. Giorgetti et al., "Interactions Between Innate Immunity, Microbiota, and Probiotics," 501361; Stephanie Collins and Gregor Reid, "Distant Site Effects of Ingested Prebiotics," *Nutrients* 8, no. 9 (September 2016): 1-20.

170. George K. Rout et al., "Benefaction of Probiotics for Human Health: A Review," *Journal of Food and Drug Analysis* 26. No. 3 (July 2018): 927–39.

171. Collins et al., "Distant Site Effects of Ingested Prebiotics," 1–20; Rout et al., "Benefaction of Probiotics for Human Health," 927–39.

172. Cremon et al., "Pre- and Probiotic Overview," 87-92.

173. Florowska, "A Prebiotics as Functional Food Ingredients Preventing Diet-Related Diseases," 2147–55.

174. Amy M. Brownawell et al., "Prebiotics and the Health Benefits of Fiber: Current Regulatory Status, Future Research and Goals," *The Journal of Nutrition* 142, no. 5 (March 2012): 962–74.

175. Cremon et al., "Pre- and Probiotic Overview," 87-92.

176. Collins et al., "Distant Site Effects of Ingested Prebiotics," 1–20.

177. Sherry Coleman Collins, "Entering the World of Prebiotics—Are They a Precursor to Gut Health? *Today's Dietitian* 16, no 12 (December 2014): 12, https://www.todaysdietitian.com/newarchives/120914p12.shtml.

178. Bethany Cadman, "What Prebiotic Foods Should People Eat?" *Medical News Today*, accessed January 2019, https://www.medicalnewstoday.com/articles/323214.php.

179. Paulina Markowiak, Katarzyna Slizewska. "Effects of Probiotics, Prebiotics, and Synbiotics on Human Health," *Nutrients* 9, no. 6: (September 2017): 1021.

180. Ibid.

181. Ibid.

182. Ibid.

183. R. Farid, H. Ahanchian, Fr. Jabbari and T. Moghiman, "Effect of a New Synbiotic Mixture on Atopic Dermatitis on Children: A Randomized-Controlled Trial," *Iranian Journal of Pediatrics* 21, no. 2 (June 2011): 225–30.

184. Roudsari et al., "Health Effects of Probiotics on the Skin," 1219–40.

185. E. G. Lopes et al., "Topical Application of Probiotics in Skin: Adhesion, Antimicrobial and Antibiofilm in Vitro Assays," *Journal of Applied Microbiology* 122, no. 2 (February 2017): 450–61.

186. Lopes et al., "Topical Application of Probiotics in Skin," 450–61; L. C. Lew and M. T. Liong, "Bioactives from Probiotics for Dermal Health: Functions and Benefits," *Journal of Applied Microbiology* 114, no. 5 (2013): 1241–53.

187. Bob Kronemyer, "Is It Time to Regulate Probiotics in Cosmetics?" *Dermatology Times* 39, no. 8 (August 2018): 68–70.

188. Ji Hye Jeong, Chang Y. Lee and Dae Kyun Chung, "Probiotic Lactic Acid Bacteria and Skin Health," *Critical Reviews in Food Science and Nutrition* 56, no. 14 (2016): 2331–37.

189. H. Tilg and A. R. Moschen, "Food, Immunity and the Microbiome," *Gastroenterology* 148, no. 6 (May 2015): 1107–19.

190. F. Sofi F et al., "Mediterranean Diet and Health Status: An Updated Meta-Analysis and a Proposal for a Literature-Based Adherence Score," *Public Health Nutrition* 17, no. 12, (December 2014): 2769–82; C. Malagoli et al., "Diet Quality and Risk of Melanoma in an Italian Population," *Journal of Nutrition* 145, no. 8 (August 2015): 1800–1807.

191. M. Á. Martínez-González, M. S. Hershey, I Zazpe and A. Trichopoulou, "Transferability of the Mediterranean Diet to Non-Mediterranean Countries. What Is and What Is Not the Mediterranean Diet," *Nutrients* 9, no. 11 (November 2017): 1–14.

192. Martínez-González et al., "Transferability of the Mediterranean Diet to Non-Mediterranean Countries," 8–9.

193. Singh et al., "Influence of Diet on the Gut Microbiome and Implications for Human Health," 1–17.

194. L. A. David et al., "Diet Rapidly and Reproducibly Alters the Human Gut Microbiome," *Nature* 505 (January 2014): 559–63

195. G. D. Wu et al., "Linking Long-Term Dietary Patterns with Gut Microbial Enterotypes," *Science* 334, no. 6052 (October 2011):105–108.

196. Singh et al., "Influence of Diet on the Gut Microbiome and Implications for Human Health," 16.

197. F. Fava et al., "The Type and Quantity of Dietary Fat and Carbohydrate Alter Faecal Microbiome and Short-Chain Fatty Acid Excretion in a Metabolic Syndrome 'At-Fisk' Population," *International Journal of Obesity* 37, no. 2 (February 2013): 216–23.

198. Singh et al., "Influence of Diet on the Gut Microbiome and Implications for Human Health," 5.

199. M. B. Hussain, "Role of Honey in Topical and Systemic Bacterial Infections," *Journal of Alternative and Complementary Medicine* 24, no. 1 (January 2018): 15–24.

200. Singh et al., "Influence of Diet on the Gut Microbiome and Implications for Human Health," 7.

201. A. Pappas, A. Liakou and C. C. Zouboulis, "Nutrition and Skin," *Reviews in Endocrine and Metabolic Disorders* 17, no. 3 (September 2016): 443–48.

202. M. Darvin, L. Zastrow, W. Sterry and J. Lademann, "Effect of Supplemented and Topically Applied Antioxidant Substances on Human Tissue," *Skin Pharmacology and Physiology* 19, no. 5 (2006): 238–47; Skylar A. Souyoul, Katharine P. Saussy and Mary P. Lupo, "Nutraceuticals: A Review," *Dermatologic Therapy* 8, no.1 (February 2018): 5–6.

203. J. Pérez-Jiménez, V. Neveu, F. Vos and A. Scalbert. "Identification of the 100 Richest Dietary Sources of Polyphenols: An Application of the Phenolexplorer Database," *European Journal of Clinical Nutrition* 64, suppl. 3 (November 2010): S112–20.

204. N. Shapira, "Nutritional Approach to Sun Protection: A Suggested Complement to External Strategies," *Nutrition Reviews* 68, no. 2 (2010): 75–86; A. Ratz-Łyko, J. Arct, S. Majewski and K. Pytkowska, "Influence of Polyphenols on the Physiological Processes in the Skin," *Phytotherapy Research* 29, no. 4 (April 2015): 509–17.

205. J. Peterson et al., "Major Flavonoids in Dry Tea," *Journal of Food Composition and Analysis* 18 (2005): 487–501.

206. C. Ankolekar et al., "Inhibitory Potential of Tea Polyphenolics and Influence of Extraction Time Against Helicobacter Pylori and Lack of Inhibition of Beneficial Lactic Acid Bacteria," *Journal of Medicinal Food* 14, no. 11 (2011): 1321–29; M. Nakayama et al., "Antibacterial Activities of Phenolic Components from Camellia Sinensis L. on Pathogenic Microorganisms," *Journal of Food Science and Nutrition* 12, no. 3 (2005): 135–40.

207. H. C. Lee, A. M. Jenner, C. S. Low and Y. K. Lee, "Effect of Tea Phenolics and Their Aromatic Fecal Bacterial Metabolites on Intestinal Microbiota," *Research in Microbiology* 157, no. 9 (2006): 876–84.

208. M. I. Queipo-Ortuño MI et al., "Influence of Red Wine Polyphenols and Ethanol on the Gut Microbiota Ecology and Biochemical Biomarkers, " *American Journal of Clinical Nutrition* 95, no. 6 (2012): 1323–34.

209. R. Puupponen-Pimiä et al., "Antimicrobial Properties of Phenolic Compound from Berries," *Journal of Applied Microbiology* 90, no. 4 (2001): 494–507.

210. Tilg et al,. "Food, Immunity and the Microbiome," 1107–19.

211. I. Bustos et al., "Effect of Flavan-3-ols on the Adhesion of Potential Probiotic Lactobacilli to Intestinal Cells," *Journal of Agricultural and Food Chemistry* 60, no. 36 (2012): 9082–88.

212. Singh et al., "Influence of Diet on the Gut Microbiome and Implications for Human Health," 7; Aleksandra Duda-Chodak, Tomasz Tarko, Paweł Satora and Paweł Sroka, "Interaction of Dietary Compounds, Especially Polyphenols, with the Intestinal Microbiota: A Review," *European Journal of Nutrition* 54, no. 3 (2015): 325–41.

213. Singh et al., "Influence of Diet on the Gut Microbiome and Implications for Human Health," 8–10.; M. R. Prado et al., "Milk Kefir: Composition, Microbial Cultures, Biological Activities and Related Products," *Frontiers in Microbiology* 6 (2015): 1177.

214. B. Shan, Y. Z. Cai, J. D. Brooks and H. Corke, "The In Vitro Antibacterial Activity of Dietary Spice and Medicinal Herb Extracts," *International Journal of Food Microbiology* 117, no. 1 (June 2007): 112–19.

215. A. R. Vaughn AR, A. Branum and R. K. Sivamani, "Effects of Turmeric (Curcuma longa) on Skin Health: A Systematic Review of the Clinical Evidence," *Phytotherapy Research* 30, no. 8 (August 2016): 1243–64.

216. Shan et al., "The In Vitro Antibacterial Activity of Dietary Spice and Medicinal Herb Extracts,"112-19; Vaughn et al., "Effects of Turmeric (Curcuma longa) on Skin Health,"1243–64.

217. Roudsari et al., "Health Effects of Probiotics on the Skin," 1219–40; Dall'Oglio et al., "Effects of Oral Supplementation with FOS and GOS Prebiotics in Women with Adult Acne," 445–49; Jeong et al., "Probiotic Lactic Acid Bacteria and Skin Health," 2331–37.

218. Bjerre et al., "The Role of the Skin Microbiome in Atopic Dermatitis," 1272–78; Roudsari et al., "Health Effects of Probiotics on the Skin," 1219–40; Jeong et al., "Probiotic Lactic Acid Bacteria and Skin Health," 2331–37.

219. Benhadou et al., "Psoriasis and Microbiota," 47; Jeong et al., "Probiotic Lactic Acid Bacteria and Skin Health," 2331–37.

220. Kano et al., "Consecutive Intake of Fermented Milk Containing Bifidobacterium breve Strain Yakult and Galacto-oligosaccharides Benefits Skin Condition in Healthy Adult Women," 33–39; Jeong et al., "Probiotic Lactic Acid Bacteria and Skin Health," 2331–37.

221. Reygagne et a.l, "The Positive Benefit of Lactobacillus Paracasei NCC2461 ST11 in Healthy Volunteers with Moderate to Severe Dandruff," 671–80.

222. Bouilly-Gauthier et al., "Clinical Evidence of Benefits of a Dietary Supplement Containing Probiotic and Carotenoids on Ultraviolet-Induced Skin Damage," 536–43.

223. Lee et al., "Clinical Evidence of Effects of Lactobacillus plantarum HY7714 on Skin Aging," 2160–68; Im et al., "Skin Moisturizing and Antiphotodamage Effects of Tyndallized Lactobacillus acidophilus IDCC 3302," 1016–23; Jeong et al., "Probiotic Lactic Acid Bacteria and Skin Health," 2331–37.

224. Grice et al., "Topographical and Temporal Diversity of the Human Skin Microbiome," 1190–92; Maguire et al., "The Role of Microbiota, and Probiotics and Prebiotics in Skin Health," 411–21; Jeong et al., "Probiotic Lactic Acid Bacteria and Skin Health," 2331–37.

225. Christopher Wallen-Russell and Sam Wallen-Russell, "Meta Analysis of Skin Microbiome: New Link between Skin Microbiota Diversity and Skin Health with Proposal to Use This as a Future Mechanism to Determine Whether Cosmetic Products Damage the Skin," Cosmetics 4, no. 14 (2017): 1–19.

226. G. Reid et al., "Microbiota Restoration: Natural and Supplemented Recovery of Human Microbialcommunities," Nature Reviews Microbiology 9, no. 1 (January 2011): 27–38; Patricia Farris, "Skincare with Probiotics—Worth the Hype?" Dermatology Times 37, no. 9 (2016): 1–4.

227. Roudsari et al., "Health Effects of Probiotics on the Skin," 1219–40; Jeong et al., "Probiotic Lactic Acid Bacteria and Skin Health," 2331–37.

228. Lopes et al., "Topical Application of Probiotics in Skin," 450–61.

229. Najeeba Riyaz and Faiz Arakkal, "Spa Therapy in Dermatology," *Indian Journal of Dermatology, Venereology and Leprology* 77, no. 2 (2011): 128–30; M. Antonelli and Donelli, "Mud Therapy and Skin Microbiome: A Review," *International Journal of Biometeorology* 62, no. 11 (November 2018):2037–44.

230. Antonelli et al., "Mud Therapy and Skin Microbiome," 2037–44.

231. Antonelli et al., "Mud Therapy and Skin Microbiome," 2037–44; S. L. Svensson et al., "Kisameet Glacial Clay: An Unexpected Source of Bacterial Diversity," *mBio* 8, no. 3 (May 2017): 1–14; Kathryn Watson, "Dead Sea Mud; Benefits and Uses," Healthline, n.d., accessed March 2019, https://www.healthline.com/health/dead-sea-mud.

232. P. McLoone, A. Oluwadun, M. Warnock and L Fyfe, "Honey: A Therapeutic Agent for Disorders of the Skin," *Central Asian Journal of Global Health* 5, no. 1 (2016): 241.

233. J. M. Alvarez-Suarez et al., "The Composition and Biological Activity of Honey: A Focus on Manuka Honey," *Foods* 3, no. 3 (July 2014): 420–32.

234. I. Ahmad, H. Jimenez, N. S. Yaacob and N. Yusuf, "Tualang Honey Protects Keratinocytes from Ultraviolet Radiation-Induced Inflammation and DNA Damage," *Photochemistry and Photobiology* 88, no. 5 (September-October 2012):1198–1204.

235. A. R. Vaughn and and R. K. Sivamani, "Effects of Fermented Dairy Products on Skin: A Systematic Review," *Journal of Alternative and Complementary Medicine* 21, no. 7 (2015): 380–85.

236. G. Yeom et al., "Clinical Efficacy of Facial Masks Containing Yoghurt and Opuntia Humifusa Raf. (F-YOP)," *Journal of Cosmetics Science* 62, no. 5 (2011): 505–14.

237. Maguire et al., "The Role of Microbiota, and Probiotics and Prebiotics in Skin Health," 411–21.

238. M. Notay, N. Foolad, A. R. Vaughn and R. K. Sivamani, "Probiotics, Prebiotics, and Synbiotics for the Treatment and Prevention of Adult Dermatological Diseases," *American Journal of Clinical Dermatology* 18, no. 6 (December 2017): 721–32; A. Gueniche et al., "Probiotics for Photoprotection," *Dermatoendocrinology* 5, no. 1 (September 2009): 275–79.

239. Notay et al., "Probiotics, Prebiotics, and Synbiotics for the Treatment and Prevention of Adult Dermatological Diseases," 721–32; Kang et al., "Antimicrobial Activity of Enterocins from Enterococcus Faecalis SL-5 Against Propionibacterium Acnes, the Causative Agent in Acne Vulgaris, and Its Therapeutic Effect,"101–109.

240. Notay et al., "Probiotics, Prebiotics, and Synbiotics for the Treatment and Prevention of Adult Dermatological Diseases," 721–32; Seite et al., "Skin Sensitivity and Skin Microbiota," 1061–64.

241. Notay et al., "Probiotics, Prebiotics, and Synbiotics for the Treatment and Prevention of Adult Dermatological Diseases," 721–32; Bjerre et al., "The Role of the Skin Microbiome in Atopic Dermatitis," 1272–78; Roudsari et al., "Health Effects of Probiotics on the Skin," 1219-1240.

242. Notay et al., "Probiotics, Prebiotics, and Synbiotics for the Treatment and Prevention of Adult Dermatological Diseases," 721–32; Fahlén et al., "Comparison of Bacterial Microbiota in Skin Biopsies from Normal and Psoriatic Skin," 15–22; Tett et al., "Unexplored Diversity and Strain-Level Structure of the Skin Microbiome Associated with Psoriasis"; Benhadou et al., "Psoriasis and Microbiota," 47.

243. Notay et al., "Probiotics, Prebiotics, and Synbiotics for the Treatment and Prevention of Adult Dermatological Diseases," 721–32; Ní Raghallaigh et al., "The Fatty Acid Profile of the Skin Surface Lipid Layer in Papulopustular Rosacea," 279–87; Grice et al., "Topographical and Temporal Diversity of the Human Skin Microbiome," 1190–92; Maguire et al., "The Role of Microbiota, and Probiotics and Prebiotics in Skin Health," 411–21.

244. Notay et al., "Probiotics, Prebiotics, and Synbiotics for the Treatment and Prevention of Adult Dermatological Diseases," 721–32; Saxena et al., "Comparison of Healthy and Dandruff Scalp Microbiome Reveals the Role of Commensals in Scalp Health," 346; Reygagne et al., "The Positive Benefit of Lactobacillus Paracasei NCC2461 ST11 in Healthy Volunteers with Moderate to Severe Dandruff," 671–80.

245. Weyrich et al., "The Skin Microbiome," 268–74.

246. M. Coleman et al., "Microbiota and Dose Response: Evolving Paradigm of Health Triangle.," *Risk Analysis* 38, no. 10 (October 018): 2013–28.

247. H. Zheng et al., "Chlorophyllin Modulates Gut Microbiota and Inhibits Intestinal Inflammation to Ameliorate Hepatic Fibrosis in Mice," *Front Physiology* 4, no. 9 (December 2018):1 671.

248. C. Callewaert et al., "Bacterial Exchange in Household Washing Machines," *Frontiers in Microbiology* 8, no. 6 (December 2015): 1381; P Prescott et al., "The Skin Microbiome," 1–16.

249. B. Abbasi et al., "The Effect of Magnesium Supplementation on Primary Insomnia in Elderly: A Double-Blind Placebo-Controlled Clinical Trial," Journal of Research in Medical Sciences 17, no. 12 (December 2012): 1161–69.

Index

~~~

Acne, 28, 32, 47, 53–56; and diet, 48; and pollution, 39, 41; and stress, 10–11; supplements, 103–104

Acne exposome, 53–54

Acne vulgaris, 32, 53–56. *See also* Acne

Actinobacteria, 26

Adaptogenic herbs, 15

Adrenal fatigue, 10

Aging. *See* Photo aging; Skin aging

Alcohol, 13. *See also* Wine

Algae. *See* Microbes

Amoxicillin, 44

Anthocyanins, 15

Antibiotics, 43, 44, 54

Antioxidants, 20–21, 94–96

Antiseptics, overuse, 43–44

Apocrine glands, 24

Arginine, 28

Atopic dermatitis, 31, 56–60; and stress, 10; supplements, 104

Avocado-Miso Dressing, 143

Azithromycin, 44

B vitamins, 16, 97

Bacteria, on skin, 2–3, 5, 21–22, 25, 26–29. *See also* Microbes; Skin microbiome

Bacteroidetes, 27

Baked Salmon with Pesto, 142

Balsamic Vinaigrette Dressing, 145

Basil, 100

"Beauty from within" concept, 19, 20, 86

Beauty wellness facts, 150, 151, 152, 153

Berries, deep-colored, 14–15

Beverages, fermented, 97

Bifidobacterium, 52, 66, 117

Biodiversity, 35–36

"Biodiversity hypothesis," 36

Bioflavonoids, 18

Bio-individuality, 88

"Biome cloud" concept, 35–36

Biome-Purifying and Detox Broth, 149

Biome-Purifying Tonic, 148

Black pepper, 101

Black tea, 102

Blackheads, 32

Blemishes, 28, 32. *See also* Acne

Blood sugar "spikes," 94

"Body burden" concept, 8

Body odor, 24, 27

Bone Broth, 147

Bone broths, 5, 102, 132; recipe, 147

"Brain-skin" axis. *See* Gut-brain-skin axis/connection

Broths, 5, 102, 132; recipes, 147, 149

Burnout, and stress, 10

Caffeine, 13

Calm app, 136

Carbohydrates, 93–94, 127

Cell phones, and digital rays, 38–39

Cereal grains, 77

Cheese, 98

Chromium, 16

Cilantro, 100

Cinnamon, 100

Clarifying Smoothie, 151

Clay therapy, 110–11

"Clean beauty" concept, 46, 107–108

Cleansers, 120, 135

Clothing alert, 135

Clove, 99

Collagen, 20; supplements, 129–30

Colony-forming units (CFU), and probiotics, 69, 73

Comfort foods, 13

Complementary ingredients, in skincare products, 118

Computers, and digital rays, 38–39

Coriander seeds, 100

Corticotropin-releasing hormone (CRH), 11

Cortisol, 10, 11

Corynebacterium, 28

Cosmetics, 45–47, 121; database, 45. *See also* Skincare

Cultured vegetables, 98–99

Cumin, 100

Dandruff, 32, 60–61; supplements, 104

Demodex mites, and rosacea, 62

Dermis (middle skin layer), 23, 24

Diet, and nutrition, 8, 13–18, 47–48, 88–106, 125–26; chart, 16–18

Dietary fiber, in fruits/vegetables, 52–53, 77, 93. *See also* Prebiotics

Digestive system, 3, 8

Digital rays, 38–39

Dirty dozen, cosmetics/chemicals, 46–47

Disinfectants, overuse, 43

DNA damage, and UV exposure, 39

Docosahexaenoic acid (DHA), 15

Dressings, salad, 141, 143, 145

Dry brushing, 136

Dry skin environment, 26

Dysbiosis (microbial imbalance), 5, 7, 9 110; acne vulgaris, 32; atopic dermatitis, 31, 56–57; avoiding, 29–33; chart, 30; sensitive skin, 33; skin microbiome, 30

Eczema, 56–58; and stress, 10; supplements, 104

Eicosapentaenoic acid (EPA), 15
80/20 rule, 88
Epidermis (outermost skin layer), 23, 24–25
Erythrasma (skin condition), 28
Exercise routine, 137
Exfoliants, 120
Exposomes, 34–35; acne, 53–54

Fats, dietary, 92–93, 128
Fatty acids, 15, 17
Fennel, 100
Fermented foods and beverages, 14, 96–99, 128
Fiber, dietary. *See* Dietary fiber
Fibroblasts, 24
"Fight or flight" concept, 10
Firmicutes, 27
Flavonoids, 95–96
Fortifying Skin, Hair and Nails Smoothie, 152
Free radicals, and aging, 20, 94
Fructo-oligosaccharides (FOS), 75
Fruits, 77, 89, 96, 127
Fungi. *See* Microbes

Galacto-oligosaccharides (GOS), 75
Gardening, 137–39
Garlic, 101
Ginger, 101
Ginger root tea, 103
"Get Your Greens" Salad with Beets and Avocado-Miso Dressing, 143
"Glo" and Go Smoothie, 152

Green tea, 102–103
Greens, 14, 102. *See also* Vegetables
Grilled Salmon and Vegetables, 146
Gut-brain-skin axis/connection, 5–18
Gut microflora, 9

Hand sanitizers, 43–44
Hand washing, 42–43
Headspace app, 136
Hemp Seed Pesto, 142
Herbs, adaptogenic, 15
Herbs and spices, 99–101, 128
Honey, 93, 112
"Hope in a jar" concept, 86
Human microbiome, in general, 1, 2, 5, 6. *See also* Gut-brain-skin axis/connection
Human Microbiome Project (HMP), 2
Hyaluronic acid, 81
"Hygiene hypothesis," 36, 41–45
Hypodermis (innermost skin layer), 23, 24
Hypothalamic-pituitary-adrenal (HPA) axis, 10

Inulin, 52–53, 75

Juices, 101–102; recipe, 150

Katz, Linda, and probiotics, 81–82
Kefir, 97
Keratin, 23, 81

Keratinocytes, 24–25
Kimchi, 98
Kimchi Omelet Anytime of the
 Day, 145
Kitchen, restocking, 127–28
Kombucha, 97; tea, 103

Labels: prebiotics, 118; probiotics,
 69–70, 73, 84, 116–18
Lacto-fermented foods, 128. *See
 also* Fermented foods and
 beverages
Lactobacillus, 51, 59, 62, 66, 117
Langerhans cells, 23
Laundry alert, 135
Leaky gut syndrome, 5, 7, 9, 47
Lederberg, Joshua, 5, 23
Legumes, 77
Lemon-Herb Vinaigrette
 Dressing, 141
"Life protection factor," 35
Lifestyle: and beauty biome,
 122–39; and skin microbiome,
 34–48
Lipoteichoic acid, 81
Low-FODMAP diet, 77–78
Luminous Skin and Antioxidant
 Smoothie, 150

Mack, Milton H., 47
Macronutrients, 91–96
Magnesium, 17; as sleep aid, 137
Makeup. *See* Cosmetics
Malassezia fungi, and rosacea, 62
Manganese, 16
Masks: body, 115; facial, 113–14,
 121, 134; recipes, 113, 134–35;

mud, 134; variations, 114;
 yogurt, 113, 134–35
Mast cells, 11
Meals: size, 14; suggestions,
 130–31. *See also* Diet and
 nutrition
Mediterranean diet, 89–91, 95
Medications, topical/internal,
 overuse, 43
Melanocytes, 23
Microbes, 1–5, 6–7, 22; inter-re-
 lationships, 37–38; and
 nutrition, 85–106; and skin-
 care, 107–21. *See also* Dysbiosis
Microbiome testing, 124–25
Microbiomes, human, 1, 2, 5, 6
Milks, 128
Minerals, 16, 17, 18, 21. *See also
 specific minerals*
Miso, 97
Mites. *See* Demodex mites
Mobile phones, and digital rays,
 38–39
Moist skin environment, 26
Moisturizers, 120–21, 135
Mud masks, 134
Mud therapy, 110, 111–12

Natto, 98
Natural mud therapy, 110, 111–12
Neubart, Melissa, 130
Nitrobacter, 117–18
Nourishing Mask with Probiotics
 and Honey, 113–14
Nutricosmetics, 19, 20
Nutrition. *See* Diet and nutrition
Nuts and seeds, 77, 128

Oils, dietary, 128
Oligofructose, 52–53
Omega-3 fatty acids, 15, 17
Oregano, 100
Organic acids, 81

Pepper, black, 101
Personal care products. *See*
  Cosmetics
pH of skin, 43
Photo aging, 61–62
Pickles, 98
Pimples, 28, 32. *See also* Acne
Pink Hair and Scalp clay mask,
  121
Pitted keratolysis (bacterial
  infection), 28
Pollution, 20, 39–41
Polyphenols, 94–96
Postbiotics, 74
Potassium, 17
Prebiotic fiber, 93. *See* Prebiotics
Prebiotics, 50—51, 52–53, 75–84;
  labeling, 118; properties,
  76–77; and skin, 53–63, 78,
  80–84; sources, 14, 75–77;
  supplements, 103–104; topical,
  78, 108–109
Probiotic metabolites, 74, 76, 81,
  91, 118
Probiotics, 12–13, 50–52, 65–74;
  benefits, 66–67, 82; defined,
  65; dosage, 73; labeling, 69–70,
  73, 84, 116–18; production,
  71–72; regulating, 68–69,
  83–84; safety, 74; shelf life,
  71–72, 84; and skin, 53–63,
67–68, 73, 80–84, 115; storage,
  74; supplements, 103–104;
  topical, 108–109
Produce, 127. *See also* Fruits;
  Vegetables
Propionibacterium, 28. *See also*
  Acne
Proteins, dietary, 14, 21, 91–92, 127
Proteobacterium, and psoriasis,
  27, 31
Psoriasis, 31, 58–59; supplements,
  104
Puberty, 22, 28

Quinoa with Red Peppers, 141

Reactive (sensitive) skin, 59–60;
  supplements, 104
Recipes: food, 141–52; masks,
  113–14, 134 –35
Red wine, 95
Resident microorganisms, on
  skin, 26
Rohlfsen, Mike, gardening tips,
  137–39
Rooibos tea, 103
Rosacea, 62–63; supplements, 104
Rosemary, 101

Savory Roasted Chickpeas, 144
Scalp, itchy. See Dandruff
Seaweed, 14
Sebaceous (oil) glands, 24; and
  dandruff, 60; skin environ-
  ment, 26, 28
Seeds and nuts, 77, 128

Sensitive skin, 33. *See* Skin, sensitive

Skin, in general: cell cycle, 11, 23; environments, 26–27; illustrations, 24, 25; layers, 23, 24, 86; mast cells, 11; microorganisms, 26; pH, 43; sensitive, 33, 59–60, 104; structure, 23–24. *See also* Gut-brain-skin axis/connection

Skin aging, 34–35; exposome, 34–35; and free radicals, 20; supplements, 104; UV rays, 61–62

Skin barrier function, 29, 40–41, 56

Skin Deep Cosmetic Database, 115

Skin microbiome, 3–4, 19–33; and lifestyle, 34–48; and nutrition, 13–18, 47–48

Skin microflora, 11, 25–29

Skincare guidelines, 119–21

Sleep, 137

Smartphones, and digital rays, 38–39

Smoothies, 14, 101–102, 129; recipes, 150–52

Soaps, overuse, 43

Soothing and Moisturizing Probiotic Mask, 134–35

Spa treatments, 135–36

Sphingomyelinase, 81

Spices and herbs, 99–101, 128

Spring waters therapy, 110, 111

Squames, 25

Staphylococcus, 27–28, 29, 43–44, 57, 60

Stratum corneum, 23–24, 25, 36–38

Streptococcus, and psoriasis, 31

Stress, 7, 136; and stress levels, 9–13; acute, 12; and the brain, 6, 9–12; charts, 12, 16–18; chronic, 12; habitual, 10; and nutrition, 13–18

Stress hormones, 10, 11

Sugar, 13

Sun protection factor (SPF), 35

Sweat and sweating, 27, 135

Sweeteners, artificial, 93

Symbiosis (balance with host), 2, 7, 27, 30, 41–42

Synbiotics, 55, 78–80, 108–109

Talib, Nigma, 3

Teas, 102–103, 128

Tempeh, 98

Tests, microbiome, 124–25

Thyme, 100

"Toasted skin syndrome," 39

Tonics, 102; recipe, 148

Transient microorganisms, on skin, 26

Tryptophan, 14

Turmeric, 100

Urbanization, 35–36

UV exposure, 20, 38–39, 61–62

van Leeuwenhoek, Antonie, 22

Vegetables, 77, 96; cultured, 98–99

Vinegars, 98–99
Vitamin A, 94
Vitamin C, 18, 94
Vitamin E, 18, 94; and pollution, 40
Vitamins, 16, 18, 21, 94. *See also specific vitamins*
Vitreoscilla filiformis, 117

Water temperature, 120
Western diet, 1, 47–48; and fats, 92; and gut, 8; and microbes, 89; and probiotics, 51

Whiteheads, 32, 53
Wild, Christopher, 34
Wine, red, 95

Yogurt-based masks, 113; recipes, 113, 134–35; variations, 114
Yogurt, dietary, 98
"You are what you eat" concept, 20, 87
Younger Skin Starts in the Gut, 3

Zinc, 18

Acknowledgments

~~~

I have to admit I was taken aback when the title idea "Good Bacteria for Healthy Skin," was brought to my attention. My initial thought was how does this even make sense? Perhaps a few years back a title like this would make absolutely no sense at all but today, with what we're learning about the microbiome, connecting bacteria to healthy skin may not be as crazy as it sounds. I've always seen things a little differently or challenged the norm, so why not write a book on bacteria for healthy skin? So, I did.

I want to thank Casie Vogel, Claire Sielaff, and the whole Ulysses Press team for finding and guiding me throughout this process. What an incredible experience.

I would like to thank my family and friends for their ongoing support and encouragement, always.

My recipe testers, Kevin and Sierra.

My Mom, who taught me how to care for my skin gently and naturally.

My Grandmother, who took me into health food stores as a child and ignited my passion for nutrition and natural health.

Ozzy, my little buddy, who sat by my side or nudged me to get outside and enjoy the outdoors.

Friends Melissa and Mike, who offered to share their expertise and wisdom.

My industry friends and colleagues, who believed in my philosophy and supported me over the years to keep moving forward. Thank you.

And for those of you that seek to see things differently. Without you we will never evolve.

About the Author

~~~

Paula Simpson is a holistic beauty expert who has integrated her expertise in biochemistry, nutrition, natural health and beauty to drive innovation within the medical, wellness and personal care sectors. With global recognition as a formulation expert for nutrition-based skincare (nutricosmetics), Paula has dedicated her time to innovating and educating both the medical aesthetic and personal care industries on the importance of nutrition to promote healthy skin and natural beauty. She has combined her scientific and holistic backgrounds to create some of the most successful nutricosmetic and beauty wellness brands available today. As a regularly sought-after natural beauty and skin nutrition expert, she has been featured on programs including *E! News*, *Entertainment Tonight*, MSNBC, *Good Morning America*, KTLA, ABC and *Fox News*, and publications like *Allure*, *Huffington Post*, *InStyle*, *Mindbodygreen*, *New Beauty Magazine*, *PopSugar*, *Reader's Digest*, *Refinery29*, *Rodale's Organic Life* and more.